The healing energies of
Trees and their Flower Essences

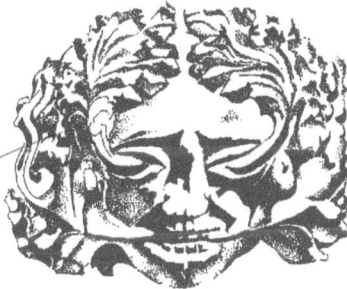

Tree Seer Publications

Tree Seer Publications

The healing energies of
Trees and their Flower Essences

ISBN 9781905454556

Design by Sue Lilly
Images by Simon Lilly

Published by:

Tree Seer Publications
'Llanddewi', Cefn Gorwydd,
Llangammarch Wells
Powys, Wales, UK, LD4 4DN
Tel: 01591 610792
Email: info@greenmanshop.co.uk
Web: www.greenmanshop.co.uk

Contents

Introduction

It was a chance remark by a student of ours that gave us the idea of tree essences. We had begun to make flower essences using the traditional methods when we moved into the Devon countryside outside Exeter. On sunny days in that first spring and summer we would collect various garden and hedgerow flowers and place them in bowls of clear water for several hours, until the water had become charged with the vibration of the plant. It was then filtered and bottled with brandy as a preservative, then stored to await assessment of its properties. We had no clear plans on working with tree essences until one evening after a lecture, someone said in passing, "Oh, I'd love to try hazel!"

Although a few tree essences had been used for many years, particularly those originally identified by Dr. Edward Bach in the 1920's and 1930's, there were not, to our knowledge, a comprehensive collection of native British tree essences available. In fact, a few years later, we found that several essence makers around the world had begun making tree essences at about the same time that the idea had come to us.

As it was February at the time we had the spring and summer to begin work. Consulting various tree books we compiled a calendar for collecting flowers. It was going to be a very busy April and May, gradually quietening down with just the occasional collection day in late summer and autumn. Hazel was already in full flower along our lanes and so this was the first essence we made - very appropriate as hazel encourages the growth of new skills, new information and focus of mind. As the weeks went by we collected more essences and began ways of solving new problems. Finding and identifying trees was just a matter of practice, but the actual collection of flowers was not always straightforward. Finding a tree in full flower on a sunny day in a fairly quiet spot often led to the frustration of not being able to reach any of the blossoms. Once we had seen that one species was beginning to flower it was often a matter of keeping an eye open for others with reachable branches.

Few of us notice the varied and seasonal appearance of tree flowers because, apart from a few exceptions like horse chestnut and the fruit trees, many are small and inconspicuous. However, once one begins to take notice it is a wonder how it was ever possible to ignore so much going on above our heads.

Humanity's relationship with trees is as old as life itself. They are, at a most fundamental level, the cause and sustainer of our reality. Climate, atmospheric composition, geology and the formation of life on this planet are largely due to green plants, and trees in particular. They are the only means by which sunlight can be turned into matter and energy. They absorb and distribute minerals that are otherwise locked in rock and soil, so that it becomes a stable sustainer of life maintaining nutrient balance and water moisture. Trees create and maintain a viable atmosphere by locking up carbon dioxide in organic compounds whilst releasing oxygen into the air. They release water vapour, which fuels the water cycle.

It is really only in the last sixty years that the expansion of the petrochemical industry has begun to replace trees as our main resource. Buildings, furniture, tools, vehicles all relied on the versatility and flexibility of wood. Heat, light, food, shelter, protection - all proceeded from trees and tree products. However much we may now replace wood with plastic or metals it still remains the case that without the tree we cannot maintain our existence in this world. It seems unthinkable that most of us walk past the largest organism we are likely to meet in our everyday lives, beings to whom we owe our very existence, and pay them as little attention as if they were chipboard wardrobes.

As well as being mankind's major resource, trees were also revered and cared for as sacred and magical beings. It is not by chance that the image of the tree appears so often as a central symbol in cosmologies, especially as the sustainer, the nurturer, the first or original home, the means to reach other levels of existence, and the means of redemption.

A tree cannot choose its place of growth. It can only survive and flourish by adjusting its form to harmonise with the prevailing conditions. The very fact that a tree grows up, matures, flowers and bears fruit means that it has succeeded in maintaining that balance for tens, hundreds, even thousands of years. It is this quality to remain balanced and flexible, to absorb and let go, to simply remain harmless that is so often transferred to tree essences.

Each species shows different habits and characteristics that are the outward, visible manifestation of the energy with which they are formed. It is the pattern of this energy that is imprinted on water molecules in the process of preparing the essences. This is why the ancient Doctrine of Signatures can still be relevant in identifying the properties of each particular tree. The Doctrine simply recognises that the outward form reflects in some way the inner energies, in a similar way that a crystal's shape is determined by the energy patterns of its constituent atoms. There is, so the Doctrine says, a symbolic significance to any resemblance, be that shape or colour or habit, that creates a resonance in a similar structure or pattern within us. Physics has discovered that there is definitely something connecting like forms that goes beyond everyday understanding of time and space. But even if we think of the Doctrine of Signatures as a constructed mnemonic system, as some researchers do, designed to associate plants with their medicinal usefulness, rather than a God-given clue to help mankind, it can still be valuable. When we have assessed our tree essences to discover their properties it is often interesting to look back at the physical characteristics, folklore and traditions. Very often there is a unifying thread of experience running through all the diverse sources.

One of the primary things we wanted to emphasise with our tree essences is that they are not just another alternative to seek out when disease symptoms pop up, as if they were an etheric or spiritual aspirin. Although they have proved to be very effective healing tools for deep level healing, we see them as a timely means for us to get back into a constructive relationship with the world through tree energies. This is why our range of essences was called *Green Man Tree Essences*. The image of the Green Man is the perfect blending of human and plant features represented for many centuries in churches and cathedrals as the ever-present power of Nature and of an underlying sense of a mysterious awareness that abides beyond the world of humans. Perhaps the closest we may now come to feeling that sense of mystery for ourselves is to walk alone into an ancient woodland or forest where, after a little while, we begin to feel a difference, a sense of otherness all around us. By integrating the vibration of trees into our own energy systems we can, perhaps, begin to experience a larger view of life, and behave with more maturity and consideration as co-creators of our world.

The active ingredient of vibrational essences is the vibration or energy pattern itself, which is essentially non-physical. Because they stimulate our subtle energy fields it is only necessary to bring the tree essence into the aura for it to begin working. For example, a few drops can be added to bathwater or into a massage oil. It can be placed on the wrist pulses, the forehead, the soles of the feet or on meridian and acupuncture points. Tree essences can be mixed with a little water, put in a diffuser spray or atomiser, and sprayed around the body or in a whole room. This is one of our favourite methods as it instantaneously infuses a new energy into any environment and is like walking into a grove of your familiar trees. We know of meditation groups who place a bowl of water containing a tree essence in their room. Each person when they enter rubs a little of the water on their hands and then passes them around the body so that the vibration of the tree enters their auric field. In this way the entire group energy becomes more coherent and had a direct link to the tree and its characteristic qualities. For example, were strawberry tree to be used, a deep level of stillness would be experienced, the crown chakra would be stimulated and positive changes would be more likely to occur at fundamental levels of the self.

Using a tree essence is a quick way to link our subtle selves to the natural world. We hope tree essences will foster a deeper awareness of our inter-relatedness, and of the unity of all life. As so much disease and illness begins from a blocking of life-force within us, or from the denial of some part of existence, it is no wonder that tree essences can be of use in the healing process and in the deepening of meditation experiences and self-discovery.

Tree Essences

In our work with trees, tree spirits and Tree Spirit Healing we have found the use of tree essences invaluable. They are, for us, one of the primary keys to open awareness to the Tree Kingdoms. Through an essence we can instantly access the energy signature, the feel, the presence and the awareness of a particular type of tree. The whole environment can become imbued with this energy and we can immerse ourselves within it.

With the physical presence of a tree, no matter how sentient or how powerful, it can be difficult for many of us to quickly go beyond the constant awareness of *selfness* that immediately sets up a subject-object relationship. This duality can create a sense of division between ourselves and the spirit worlds. We are used to our physical existence, the presence of our bodies and of being inside them. We always look out, and so are separated from the world. Whatever is out there belongs to the realm of the five senses and when we begin to perceive or understand something that seems outside of the sense organs it is very easy to doubt the experience. It very easily becomes downgraded to 'only our imagination'.

Using tree essences we can help to remove this perceptual and intellectual barrier. Not only can we step into the energy of a tree, for example, when the essence is sprayed around the room, but the tree energy can directly enter into us if a few drops are taken by mouth, or rubbed into the pulse points. In other words, using a tree essence helps to amplify the experience of the characteristic feel of a tree. Not only do we perceive with our external senses the quality of a physical tree, but we activate all our internal senses as well - those feelings and body wisdom mechanisms that in everyday, externalised life we tend to ignore.

There seems to be no clear historical evidence of the use of flower essences as we recognise them today, though there are similar, subtle techniques described in a wider cultural context. The most apparent seems to be the collection of morning dew, off flowers and leaves, recorded in medieval European magical traditions. Paracelsus in the 16th century is reputed to have done this to heal emotional imbalances in his patients. As he seems to have been an important synthesiser of Classical and native European (pagan) healing and spiritual techniques, it is reasonable to assume that he was borrowing from already established sources. When Dr. Edward Bach first started his experiments with flower energies in the 1920's he seems to have combined the magical dew-collecting of Paracelsus with the theoretical background of homoeopathy. With direct personal intuitive insights he began by roaming the countryside at dawn collecting and drinking the dew off certain plants. For practical reasons he developed other collecting and preparation techniques that are still in use by flower essence makers today.

Among the native peoples of the world, flowers and plants are the primary source of healing and spiritual energies. As the power of the plant is believed to come from its spirit, many cultures will include preparations from the required plants by making broths, baths, bundles, oils, tinctures and so on, to be administered externally or internally. The chemical properties of the plant may or may not be employed in a conscious manner - it is the spirit is all-important. We shall see that in modern flower essence usage, subtracting all the jargon and pseudo-scientific terminology, it also comes back to the same thing: the intangible, indefinable, unmeasurable spirit of the plant.

So what is a flower essence? A flower essence is an energy signature of a plant held in water, usually preserved in brandy or another alcohol. Orthodox testing would reveal nothing other than water and brandy. There is no physical presence of the plant at all. In this way, flower essences differ from that other more well-known energy medicine, homoeopathy, where at lower potencies there can still be found minute amounts of original material.

Just about the only tangible evidence that something subtle is going on in a flower essence, can be revealed by taking a Kirlian photograph of an essence droplet and comparing them to other essences, to plain water or alcohol. The energy discharge from an essence is immediately recognisable by its dynamism and corona. However, the most sensitive apparatus

Making an Essence

If you want to make an essence, begin by using the most straightforward sun and water method. Once familiar with the process you will be more confident to modify and try other approaches.

1. Get a plain glass bowl that, if possible, is free of all patterns, names and numbers. (These will carry their own vibration so it is best to avoid confusing your essence). Some better class of glassware has removable labels, and inexpensive dessert bowls are often free from stamping. If you are thinking of making a few essences, you may want to have bowls of different sizes. This is because it is best to cover the whole surface of the water with flowers and, while some flowers are quite large, others including a lot of tree flowers, are very small.

2. You will need to fill this bowl with as pure a water as possible. Spring water is the best, direct from the source if possible, or else use a good quality bottled water. It is not really possible to avoid pollutants these days, even groundwater may have high levels of chemical fertiliser.

3. It is best to make essences only of those plants that attract your attention, that draw you in some way to them. These are plants with which you have some significant link at that time, so you will automatically be more in tune with their energy patterns.

4. Spend some time familiarising yourself with the tree or plant. This doesn't necessarily mean sitting for hours boring the spirits with doe-eyed mood-making, unless you like that sort of thing. It is best to have some heart connection with the plant's presence, but it is very unlikely that you will have no empathy or you would have no interest in this sort of thing in the first place.

5. If the essence is to be of a tree flower and you know the attuning techniques that we have developed, you can use the appropriate ones to create a more substantial flow of energy between you.

6. When you feel comfortable with the plant's presence (this may be almost immediate or can be a slow growth of appreciative awareness over a week or two), it is a good idea to verbally or mentally explain what you are going to do and for what reasons.

7. Also ask permission to take flowers from the plant. The emotional intent of harmlessness and sensitivity are very obvious to plant awareness so coherent framing of thought is more important for your own clarity of purpose than to the plant. Clarity of thought may also help you to focus you're emotional/feeling stance.

8. When you ask for permission it is important to quieten your mind and listen or feel for a response. This you might perceive as an inner voice or as a change of emotional pressure, either relaxing or tensing. If you feel resistance in some way, ask again and if the feeling remains the same move to another plant or try again some other time. If communication is good you might try ask what is the reason for the refusal. Sometimes it can be just a simple question of etiquette, or you may need to perform some small ritual act to get into a more appropriate state of mind. If it is the tree itself that is unwilling to participate, finding out why can sometimes allow you to help by offering healing. A genuine offering of assistance is never wasted- even though you might have to modify your thought patterns to elicit a positive response. Some tree spirits can be very tetchy if they have suffered in the past from lack of care or are unwell.

9. When you have felt the positive response to your request to take a few flowers, you can go about carefully collecting them. If possible it is a good idea to collect flowers from different parts of the tree or from different nearby trees. What you are able to reach will somewhat limit this choice as not all trees put out flowers near to the ground. Looking out for trees growing on slopes will become an automatic pastime, where more of the mature branches can be reached. How you pick the flowers is up to you and you will need to experiment with different methods until you find one that is comfortable for you. I find that different trees require different techniques simply because of the physical diversity of flowers. Some are easy to pinch off without crushing them using a pair of silver sugar tongs, others need more dexterous fingers and sharp nails to gather. Many tree flowers are very small and you will need a degree of focused patience as well as a relatively small bowl.

10. As you collect the flowers place them carefully on the surface of the water. When there are enough to cover the surface, leave the bowl in full sun close to the plant. Sometimes it will not be possible to leave the bowl, so if this is the case just place the bowl on some kind of natural surface, such as wood or stone (try to avoid the strong unnatural vibration of metal, plastic or concrete).

11. Take care where you place the bowl. What starts off in full sun, may in a short time be in deep shade and this will lengthen the energising process. Also, if you are leaving the bowl for any length of time be aware of the possibility that it will be found by domestic animals - thirsty dogs and curious cats can demolish a day's work in a moment, so place the bowl high enough off the ground.

12. The length of time it takes to energise the water is very variable. Different essence-makers use many different rules and regulations, but what is laid down in one book may not be the most useful technique for you to use. So much depends on the conditions when the essence is being made. Classically, the optimal time for essence-making is in the early morning in spring or summer time on a cloudless, sunny day. In these conditions two or three hours is often cited as being sufficient to potentize the water. Since many books on essences are written by Americans who live on the West Coast of the USA, adverse weather conditions are rarely considered. Compared to the British Isles, southern California has no weather: when the sun is not shining, it is night-time. Clouds, six different climates in an hour, and startlingly short flowering periods coinciding with weeks of continuous rain -that is the norm for the British essence maker. It has the tendency to create jumpy, nervous individuals who continually glance from bud to sky to bud again, but it also creates flexibility, opportunism and new ways of working. The only rule you need in essence making is: do what is appropriate at the time, according to your insight.

13. In conditions that are less than ideal, when there is cloud cover, or if you expect sunshine and showers, allow longer exposure of the essence to sunlight. In really dull conditions you might consider putting the bowl on a mirror surface to reflect the light. On rainy days cover the bowl with a sheet of glass or a larger bowl to prevent swamping with rain water. Use your imagination and experiment. If you have been inspired to make an essence at a certain time, make it then. It will be the most powerful for you whatever the conditions.

14. It is important whenever possible to use flowers that are in full bloom and undamaged. This very often means carefully watching your chosen tree for the best time to prepare the essence. You will find that trees of the same species will flower at different times depending on their age and where they are situated. If you find your tree has already passed its peak and is dropping petals, look around for another tree that has slightly later flowering. Remember that different parts of the same tree will often be ahead or behind the rest in its growth cycle depending whether it is in sun or shade.

15. If you don't have a testing skill like dowsing or muscle-testing you will have to rely more on the rules, or else quieten yourself and ask your deep mind or intuition to let you know when the essence 'feels' ready to bottle.

16. Essences made at any time of year except very early in spring or late autumn will tend to accumulate at least a few insects, as well as wind-blown sticks and leaves. These will have to be lifted out of the water together with the flowers. What you do with these flowers is up to you, but it is important to treat them with care and consideration. They can be dried to use as a basis for incense, offerings, herb bundles; placed in another decorative bowl as an indoor display until they fade; placed back under the trees you have gathered from; put on the soil or in compost to continue the cycle of life.

17. Whatever you do, do it with awareness and thanks. Some authors suggest a twig or leaf of the plant is used to lift the flowers off the water. Try it and see: sometimes it works, sometimes it is far too awkward.

Avoid frustration if at all possible. It is a strong projecting emotion and can interfere with the quality of your essence. A small silver spoon or silver sugar tongs are quite versatile and silver is a fairly benign, neutral metal to use.

18. Once the flowers and larger bugs are removed it is a good idea to filter out smaller particles of flower, pollen and creepy-crawlies. Using another clean glass vessel strain the water through a fine cheesecloth, linen or filter paper. This will help to prevent any fungal or bacterial growth in the essence bottle.

19. Most essence makers use a spirit such as brandy or vodka for a preservative. If alcohol is a problem, a vinegar will preserve equally effectively, though the smell and taste tends to linger long after the alcohol would have evaporated. Fill the storage bottle at least half-full with the preservative and then top up with the potentized water. Give the mix a good shake to help the stabilisation of the energies. This is now the mother essence. Clearly label and date it. Most essence makers will keep the mother essence as the primary source and will use the dilution commonly called the stock bottle. Stock is made by taking a few drops, usually between three and seven, from the mother essence and putting them in another bottle containing at least fifty percent brandy and topped up with water.

20. Whether you use the mother essence or the stock essence (or even the next dilution down-the 'dosage' level where drops are taken from the 'stock' and placed in another bottle of water/brandy), will depend on how much essence was originally made and how frequently it is going to be used.

Each essence maker seems to have their own ideas concerning the efficacy of the different levels of dilution. We suspect most are adhering to a set of personal belief-systems with which they feel comfortable (and therefore effective in their own experience), rather than there being one ineffable law of nature entitled: "Essences and the Uses Thereof." We return to the original perplexity. What is it that comprises an essence? If it is essentially a physical process then it should be able to be measured in some way. If it is not a physical process then the rules of mass, weight, proportion, location in time and space, and other means of measuring the 'amount' of essence present in any one bottle cannot apply. If this is so, then how can one dilute a vibration that has no mass etc. It is either there or not there. It is difficult to conceive of an energy pattern that is 'not-there-very-much'.

Being human, however, precise measurement, the process and the recipe - all the ritual of creating and passing on information and knowledge - is very important to most of us. Following instructions means that we know when we are right and when we have done it wrong. Doing the same thing as someone else who has got a good result makes us likely to encourage a similar outcome, and so it will tend to happen that way. "Take three drops, four times a day and you will get better" is what the majority of us want to hear. We don't like to be reminded of self-responsibility and self-determination. Most of us haven't been trained to really understand what these qualities mean. "Do as you're told" has been endlessly reinforced through the long years of schooling. Whilst "Do what you think is best" often seems suspiciously like the precursor of avoiding or attributing blame.

Alternate Methods of Making Essences
It is well worth making a few tree essences for yourself, firstly to establish the ease of the process and, secondly, to experience the nuances and shifts of awareness that occur during the whole time. There is a particular state that soon descends as one goes out with the intention to make a flower essence. It feels very close to meditative states and the heightened awareness achieved during intensive retreats. The simplicity and tried and tested efficacy of the traditional sun-water method should be used first of all.

Over the years new methods have evolved that seem to prove equally effective and provide solutions in instances where the sun-water method may be inappropriate. These new techniques slide effortlessly away from any scientifically justifiable procedures and simply become akin to magical invocation and evocation.

The early essence maker, Dr Edward Bach, was flexible in his approach. Although the sun-water technique arose from the early dew-drinking phase, a good proportion of his flower essences were prepared by boiling. Now boiling, can, in no way, be understood as a simple vibrational technique. The result will always be a herbal infusion or tisane of some concentration. It can still be argued that the energy signature is also present in the water, but there will be quite a physical molecular presence as well. And what can be said of the remedy Rock Water? Rock Water is exactly what it says it is - water collected from mountain streams running through and over native rock. It does what it says, but there is not a flower in sight. Today there are an increasing number of such 'environmental essences' that have been made to capture a particular time or place. There are essences of locations, equinoxes, sacred sites, specific types of environments, sea creatures, dolphins, whales, planets and stars. All have, in some way, encapsulated the unique energy of the 'target' but none can use the sun-water method as developed and promoted by Dr. Bach.

The first group of essences that we heard about that used one of these new methods was a collection of Amazonian orchids. When you are dealing with rare or endangered species collecting a bowl full of blooms would be an environmentally unsound practice. And, considering the flowers might appear several hundred feet up in the tree canopy, dotted here and there throughout the rainforest, it would also be a logistic nightmare to undertake. The solution in this instance was to employ the energies of a quartz crystal as an intermediary, where the perfect lattice structure of the quartz surrogates for the flexible lattice of water, and in some way, receives the energy signature of the plant for a later transference back into water.

We have now come across and used many different methods of essence making. For instance, the flower or flowers can be left unpicked and simply bent gently down until they contact the surface of the water in the bowl.

Or, more cunningly, a container can be attached to the plant where, for a short period of time, flowers can be held in the water. We saw an ingenious and elegant alchemical device that carefully held the flower in a sealed chamber whilst spring water dripped over it and was collected in a lower chamber. Instead of a bowl of glass some essence makers use beautiful hollow geodes of crystal. Quartz being an extremely sensitive material, it reacts very strongly to intention and so can focus the correct or appropriate energy very accurately into the water it contains. One of the most powerful essences we have ever tried was made by simply placing a clear quartz crystal close to a group of Monterey Cypresses on the California coastline. The essence maker had intended to place the crystal in a fork of the tree but was firmly persuaded by the tree itself to simply place the stone at the base of its trunk. The crystal was then placed in water and the energy pattern transferred to the liquid.

It is also possible to make an essence without any process or intervention at all, except for the focused intention of the maker and the willing co-operation of the plant spirit in question. A sealed bottle already prepared with brandy and water can be left in or close to the plant for a specific length of time and the spirit itself infuses or imprints the water. The less involved we become in the making, the more attention will need to be given to the exact requirements of the target plant. Is it best to use a crystal, crystal and water, open water, sealed water, sealed water with brandy, pure brandy? And so on. Also what time of exposure will be needed, at what time of day; the exact placement of the vessel and what is the sort of vessel to be used?

All in all, it is probably better always to go with the technique that feels most comfortable. This will be the one that creates the least turbulence at subtle levels and so will tend to allow for the making of a purer essence. Some essence makers enjoy picking the flowers by hand, feeling that it thus becomes a powerful shared process between human and plant kingdoms, whilst others prefer to leave the plants as untouched as possible. Depending on one's viewpoint of humanity's role and place on the planet, these viewpoints might seem either exploitative or apologetic.

Using Essences

Once we have an essence what can be done with it? How can it be used? Flower essences today are used almost exclusively in the area of healing. The various paradigms of flower essence therapy reflect and expand upon the original vision of Dr Bach. His selection of plant essences addressed what he considered to be the underlying negative emotional states that allowed disease to manifest in the physical body. He discovered that by some means the energy pattern of each flower encouraged the negative state to transform to its more life-supporting and positive opposite.

This view has been generally agreed and expanded upon by all recent essence makers. The specific and unique energy signature of each essence, when introduced in some way into the human auric field seems to enable positive change to come about more easily. An essence acts like a key that can unlock doors that have been shut or blocked. This is an important concept. Many believe that flower essences do not create change by themselves, but they do allow change to take place. This can be compared by analogy to a physical herbal or pharmaceutical preparation that, instead of unlocking the door leaving you free to open it or not, will carry out a full FBI raid with tanks, helicopters, hand-grenades, howitzers and CS gas blowing away anything that comes into their path be it door, wall, hostage-taker or hostage. In some health situations such action is necessary, but in the main it can be avoided by carefully stimulating the body's own healing processes. This is, ultimately, the only thing that can heal us, and flower essences seem to be very good at supporting this.

Flower essences do not work by believe or faith, nor placebo effect, because essences work extremely well on animals, small children and plants. However, their actions can sometimes be blocked by negative attitudes or environment factors. Always when working with essences (for whatever reason, healing or otherwise), a willing participation and a neutral curiosity are good attitudes to have. It is good practice to use the essences in a conscious manner. Focus for a moment on the reason you are taking the essence, whether for healing or whatever. Give the bottle a brief shake before opening.

This helps to activate and energise the properties. Visualise or otherwise acknowledge the plant's source, the spirit of the essence. Sit quietly for a moment or two as you absorb the vibrational energies into your system. Don't expect the essence to create mind-blowing altered states, instant healing, revelatory visions and so on, every time you use it. All these can happen, occasionally. More often the essences will work at much more subtle levels, creating or allowing energy changes that may take weeks or months to become noticeable. This is particularly likely when you are in a state of considerable imbalance, as with manifest physical illness.

Using a tree essence as a Tree Teacher Technique, your attention will already naturally be focused on a change of perception and will be looking out for subtle differences of feel. Using tree essences as a specific healing technique will be explored further in a later chapter.

Different Ways Of Taking Essences
The classic way of using flower essences is to take three or four drops, three times a day either placed under the tongue and held in the mouth for a little while, or placed in some water and sipped as necessary. Generally speaking, no method is better than any other - as long as the essence comes in contact with the energy field, interaction will take place. Some people will find that certain ways of introducing the essences will work faster or more effectively for them, but it is very much down to personal experience.

The advantage and disadvantage with taking by mouth is that it reinforces the comparison with taking medicine, with all the expectations and limitations that comes with such a view. Many people will not feel they have done it properly unless they stick to the old, familiar procedures. This is fine. The main disadvantage with the oral taking of essences is one of association rather than effect: it emphasises the 'just-another-thing-to-make-me-better' attitude, and this really can be quite a negative and dis-empowering, reinforcing as it does, the idea that effective healing can only come from outside of oneself. It also limits the use of flower essences to the role of 'spiritual aspirin' where the name of the essence - the actual plant, gemstone or whatever - is regarded as little more than an identifying label.

The stuff in the bottle becomes conceptually isolated from its real source, the plant energy, the living stuff. In this process there is the danger of becoming one-sided, of becoming a spiritual colonialist, simply taking over another part of the world and exploiting it in order to make ourselves 'better' without considering reciprocity.

Dr. Bach suggested that when the taking of essences by mouth was inadvisable, in instances of unconsciousness or physical trauma, they could be applied topically to the forehead or to the wrist pulses. In fact, this proves to be equally effective in most situations. The pulse points of the wrists and the neck and forehead, particularly the frontal eminences, (the slight raised bumps on the outer edge of the forehead), are very sensitive to a change of energy and seem a natural place to rub a few drops of essence. You can even pretend it's a perfume or aftershave if you're in hostile territory.

Anywhere where there is a mirroring of the whole systems of the body in a small area is a good place to put the essence. Thus the soles of the feet, the palms of the hands, and the ear lobes will all tend to activate the essence effectively.

If you are aware of your own strengths and weaknesses as far as the chakra system is concerned then putting a drop of essence on these specific areas will act as a rapid enhancer and diffuser through that system of interlinked energies. It can often be quite easy to determine our dominant chakra points: very often they are those areas that we use a lot and where we also tend to get minor health problems. Where we focus our energies is where we can be vulnerable to disorders simply because depletion can more easily occur there. Thus a communicator may be prone to sore throats, thyroid imbalance or neck problems. Someone who works with the heart chakra will be very sensitive to other people's emotions and may have vague heart and lung aches from time to time. A strong solar plexus energy may be prone to food sensitivities, stomach aches and so on. Because the seven main chakra points are in effect gateways or regulators of all our energy systems, they are, in any case, important sites for essences.

A drop of the essence on the appropriate chakra can create profound rebalancing that may otherwise take months to accomplish by other means. The chakra system has the advantage of being fairly easy to comprehend in broad terms and easy to locate on the physical body. Some essence makers who are familiar with the meridian systems of the body have done some exciting work isolating specific meridian points as sites to apply essences for particular results. The meridian system is not easy to master quickly. Unless you have an in-depth knowledge or an accurate testing procedure that you can wholly rely on, plopping essences on acupoints may have an unsettling or even unbalancing effect on the system as a whole. However, if this method appeals to you, consider working with the end-points of each meridian (usually on the hands, feet and head), which will give a general activation to the whole of that meridian.

Meridian Massage
There is a relatively simple technique known as meridian massage that, once learned, is an excellent way to tone up the whole meridian system and if you rub a few drops of essence into your hands before you begin, will carry the essence effectively through the whole system. Meridian massage can be carried out on yourself and on others.

Working on another person:

1. Start by having them stand upright, legs shoulder-width apart and arms held palms inwards, slightly away from the body.

2. Begin with both of your hands in front of their heart in the centre of the chest. Carry out all movements in easy, flowing sweeps of your hands an inch or so away from the body. Move your hands up from the heart to the armpits and down the insides of the arms to the hands.

3. Follow around their fingertips to the tops of the hands and then up the outside of the arms to the shoulders either side of the neck.

4. Move up the sides of the neck and bring your hands together under the jaw so that they then travel together over the centre of the face, up towards the top of the head.

5. Carry this sweep on down the back of the head and right down the spine. Then follow down the outside of the legs to the feet, around the toes and then sweep up the midline back to the heart.

6.If you follow this movement several times your hands and arms will have traced in a strengthening direction all the major meridian pathways.

7. Complete the process by moving round to the side of the person and move your hands from a starting point at the base of the spine at the back and near the groin at the front, sweeping both hands simultaneously up the body. The hand at the front ends and lightly touches the point just below the lower lip, and the hand at the back runs over the top of the head and touches a point just above the upper lip.

8. Repeat this 'zipping up' sweep a couple of times. This helps to stabilise and secure the meridian energy.

This simple procedure by itself, even without any essence, can make a lot of difference to energy levels and feelings of well-being. Done consciously and with focus it can sometimes have a profound effect equal to any other healing session.

Meridian massage on yourself is the same process except you have to do it bit by bit.

1.Start at the heart again. Move your left hand from heart to front of the right shoulder down inside of the right arm to the palm and fingertips.

2. Then repeat the movement on the left side with your right hand sweeping from heart to fingertips along the inside of the arm (hold your hand palm upwards to expose the correct bits of the arm).

3. Return to sweeping with your left hand, and now begin where you stopped before at your right fingertips, this time sweeping up the knuckles, wrist and top/outside of the arm around the shoulder and back over the chest to the heart. Repeat this on the other side of the body.

4. Next take both hands to the heart and sweep up your midline up the face, over the top of the head and as far down your neck or back as you can reach.

5. Taking your hands round to your back the other way (reaching back under your arms), continue to sweep down the rest of the back down the backs of your legs, around the outside edges of your feet and toes to the inside of your feet and legs moving upwards until your hands meet again at the groin, where they continue on together up the front of the body to stop at the heart. This is one circuit.

6. You can repeat it as many times as you like, always remembering to 'zip up' front and back midlines at the end of the process.

This process is much easier to do than to describe! Once the sequence is worked out it is well worth doing daily as a routine energy balance or when you are feeling disorientated or unusually strange.

The more you get used to having balanced energy the easier it is to notice when you drift out of balance, and the more awareness you will have of situations that are life-enhancing and those that are potentially life-damaging.

Meridian massage with a few drops of tree essence on the palms of the hands not only restores the balance in a general way to the energy systems, but also helps to align the individual to the specific energy signature of that essence. The rather ritual nature of the practice of meridian massage, once memorised, can become an easy way to move oneself into balanced, altered states. Whilst it defines the physical boundaries of the body, it also resembles the donning of magical clothes, the preparation to begin moving beyond.

Heat is a similar vibration Sound is a vibration of matter. Any vibration by its very nature tends to set up vibrations in the things around it. When this vibrational energy is echoed by other matter it is called 'resonance'. So, a sound made in one place sets up a resonance in the molecules of air and earth and can be heard a great distance away from its source. Each energy has certain sounds, colours, shapes with which the resonant quality is very strong, creating a coherent feedback link between them.

Resonance can be at a physical level of vibration or it can be at a subtle level of vibration. Only those things with an in-built tendency to resonate to a specific vibration will act as a resonant body. Thus our eyes have developed to recognise colour and shape, and our ears have developed to recognise sound. Subtle resonance is the skill that the human mind possesses. It can feel and discern energy links between forms that are not obvious to external observation. The unconscious mind works largely through resonance in the form of symbols. Shapes, colours and even language itself are symbolic and the mind uses these resonant forms to 'conjure up' objects, events and experiences that are not physically present. The symbols we have developed for each tree are precisely this type of symbolic resonant form that automatically help to tune the mind to the inherent core energy of the tree it represents.

To define anything in creation properly, its relationship to everything else in creation needs to be known. Names begin this process of verbal definition. A person has a given name, a family name (linking to the ancestral line), a title (defining relationship to other individuals), a job title (defining function within the society). This, however, does little to define the person as a unique individual. We cannot know from this information their likes and dislikes, who they know, what they have done in their lives, but these names, these symbolic forms, work well enough at everyday levels for others to comprehend who is being talked about, and for the person themselves to respond to any request. A name is a resonant symbol for an individual.

Working with a great many different mental techniques over more than a dozen years, we have built up a familiarity with the tree energies that have allowed us to concentrate or condense the qualities of a tree species into a series of symbolic forms that allow an automatic and continual resonance with those trees.

In the same way that a flower essence holds the vibrational pattern of a species in water, a specific shape and colour, sound (word pictures and sequences of syllables or mantra) can do the same.

Sound will create a pattern in sand that has been spread upon a resonating surface. In the same way the unique patterns of a tree species form patterns upon the sensitive layers of a receptive mind. The accuracy of the pattern will always be the same – the perception or interpretation of the pattern may well see some variations because of local influences (the energy quality of each person and their ability to transfer energy into a relevant form). A flower essence can be described as a solution for the negative emotion of jealousy. It may also be described as encouraging acceptance of self. Again the same essence might be defined as having a green energy pattern. These definitions might confuse someone who thinks that there must be only one explanation that is correct, whereas in fact all these explanations are an attempt to define, by different means, the same qualities.

The mantra

Most ancient cultures agree that sound is the primary energy of creation, that sound, the vibration of matter, creates form. Therefore to identify the sound that precisely defines a form can create resonant entrainment - the sound manifests the form on one level or another. Chants, prayers, spells, mantras, are all effective simply because their pattern of sound folds the subtle matter of the mind in such a way as to create the energy resonance of whatever is being focused upon.

The phonetic sounds that we have given here for each tree are those that, in a very abbreviated form, represent (in sounds made by the human mouth), the energy space or resonant energy of that tree species.

The visual key

The visual symbols are like a snapshot, a single camera frame, of a constantly moving, dynamic interplay within and around the tree. They have arisen within the mind during deep attunement and contemplation of each tree's core energy nature. These dynamic energy forms, or dances, have then been distilled as accurately as possible into a single two-dimensional visual shape or pattern. The colour of the visual symbol gives the main focus with which the tree energy works with human states of balance and imbalance.

The colour sequence

The energy of the tree expressed in a sequence of colours is very specific to the internal spiritual nature of the tree's own awareness. (This, then, can differ from the colouring of the visual key, which simply refers to how humans can be helped by the healing qualities of that tree.) The colour sequence represents the tree's own inherent nature irrespective of any usefulness it may have to other beings. The sequence is a means of translating the unique way that a tree species manifests particular aspects of universal energy. Sometimes the main healing colour is reflected in the spirit colour sequences, but often it is not. At the level of causes and effects those skilled in tracing how energy moves through the universe would be able to see a clear progression in how each of these vibrations interact in the world. But it is not necessary to intellectually try to interpret the colour sequences. Some broad tendencies might be deduced, but as nothing exists in isolation, there is no end to the possibilities of translating each sequence. We can content ourselves that we have the ends of a few threads that are linked in with a much greater universal fabric, a point of contact that will allow us to access the tree energy at a much deeper level.

Note Sequence

Sequences of notes have a profound effect on the mind and emotions. It is a form of communication that expresses a vast amount of information that is completely free from the restrictions of language. The note sequences we have deduced for trees can be quite elaborate or very simple. They can be used in a relaxed and playful manner. First, become familiar with the sound sequence - they can often seem awkward or strange to begin with. Feel free to experiment with the length of each note, but keep the same notes in the same order. When you become familiar with the sequence you may pick up harmonies and variations. The sequences can be played as single notes or as chords. Sometimes it is quite easy to combine the tree mantra with the note sequence, and this can be a quick way to deepen your experience of the tree energy in a meditative manner. If you don't play a musical instrument a simple inexpensive keyboard app. is a great way to get the notes right.

Common name and species name
The trees are identified by their common English name (where one exists), and its Latin botanical classification. Both are energy symbols in language form that represent the tree's energy reality in some degree. They have less power at an unconscious level that the mantra, however, because they tend to pull the attention towards outward form, rather than the core spiritual (non-physical) energy. There may also be traditional, or regional folk names that will give evocative clues to some of the qualities of the species.

The Tree Essences

In this book we have listed all our tree essences.

The qualities we have discerned and discovered about the essences are
described in non-medical terms.
 In the UK is has been illegal to use medicinal descriptions for essences
since 2005. The turning points was both a blow and a godsend. The breadth
of essences available in the UK was nearly lost due to changes in the law
regarding traditional herbal products, medicinal products and what could be
claimed as to their efficacy.
 The choice was stark. Let essences stay in the medicinal category and be
prepared to pay out huge sums of money to gain medicinal licences for each
product, or allow essences to be categorised as foods. Categorisation as
foods meant that there were to be no medicinal or medical claims made for
them and food labelling laws had to be followed.

 We started to use a shorthand for the qualities of our essences. This has
remained. We describe them in colour, chakra and meridian terms. This
shorthand can then be expanded by using basic information of colour,
chakra and meridians, (these can be found in the appendices of this book).

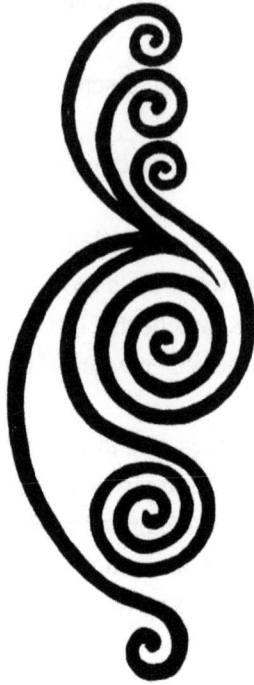

Alder *(Alnus glutinosa)*

Keyword: release

Colour: orange

Chakras: 2, 3, 4

Mantra: TISH LEE PIN O

Note Sequence: *A *G *G
(* before the notes indicates the octave below Middle C)

 Colour Sequence: white - red - green

Alder *(Alnus glutinosa)*

Alder grows throughout the British Isles along rivers and streams. The lack of oxygen in the wet soil is no problem to the tree as its roots are home to nitrogen-fixing bacteria that help to free up nutrients the alder can use. In fact the common or black alder prefers to have its dark red roots growing in a constant flow of water. These roots are a significant factor in the maintenance of our riverbanks and also increase the fertility of the soil.

The Central meridian (Conception Vessel), which provides a source of primary life-energy to the meridian system and which focuses on survival issues and self-identity, is energised. Stomach and Small Intestine meridians are also activated promoting an increase of happiness and joy.

A clarity is brought to the mind and the mental body, associated with thought processes and belief systems, is strengthened. With this cleansing of the mental body naturally related physical tensions can be eased, so that alder is useful for muscular tension that has an emotional component. (Combines well with dandelion extract or essence for relaxation).

The heart chakra and solar plexus chakra are activated. This increases the sense of well-being and life-energy available, which naturally reduces anxiety levels. Energy is able to flow from the solar plexus chakra to the heart chakra to release any energy blockages due to accumulation of stress and tension. When the heart chakra receives more energy the entire system becomes better balanced and is able to release stored stresses more easily. This may be expressed as involuntary deep breaths, sighs or crying as a means to release old wounds.

Alder provides many dyes from its parts: bark alone gives red and is the basis for black dyes, bark and young shoots give yellow and shades of orange-pink, fresh wood provides a pinkish fawn, catkins give green.

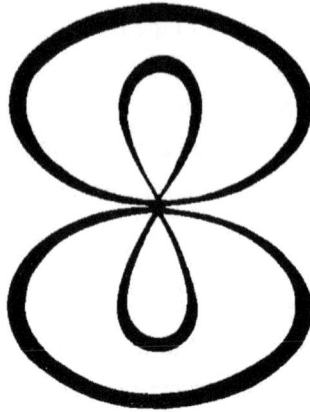

Apple *(Malus domesticus, Malus sylvestris)*

Keyword: detoxification

Colour: Orange

Chakras: 2, 4

Mantra: DOW PRRRNGAA

Note Sequence: F Eb C# F G F Eb C# C

(* before the notes indicates the octave below Middle C)

Colour Sequence: gold - green - yellow

Apple *(Malus domesticus, Malus sylvestris)*

Wild crab apple is native to Britain and is found in hedgerows and oakwoods. Wild apple has mainly white flowers and some thorns. It is one of the original species from which the sweeter, larger domestic apples were grown. Domestic apples found in gardens and orchards are also common along paths and roadsides where discarded cores have been thrown. Cross-breeding and the many varieties of apple can sometimes make exact identification difficult.

With apple there is an increased balance of purpose, a clarity and ability to express needs precisely. With this influx of discrimination it becomes apparent which aspects of life are not productive, or that are even damaging. Choices can then be made to abandon inappropriate patterns in favour of those that will allow a growth of happiness and fulfilment.

The heart chakra is greatly affected by apple's energy patterns. A cleansing and balancing of this area helps to give clarity to our spiritual direction and personal path – so apple can be used for indecision or doubt as to actions. There is a greater desire to enjoy life, to learn and make use of experiences. This can help both the timid to explore further and restrain the overly reckless from impulsive action. Perceptive insights become sharper and there is a greater access to higher states of awareness and the information that can flow from these levels.

The emotions are stabilised and directed into constructive channels whilst still maintaining a healthy lust for life. Harmony and understanding others becomes easier. Spiritual nature is opened up to wisdom, healing, a clearer understanding of self and to new areas of perception and inspiration.

In practical terms these effects strengthen the whole and speed up the removal of unwanted energies. Clarity of mind and emotions reduces tension, and this new relaxation makes spiritual energies more easily available.

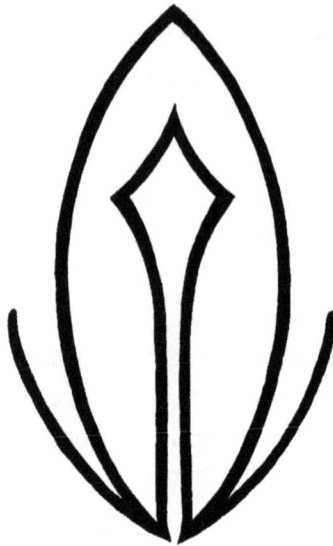

Ash *(Fraxinus excelsior)*

Keyword: strength

Colour: green

Chakra: 1, 4

Mantra: D'HAA – GAA. D'HRRRR – AA. SHRR

Note sequence: A Ab Ab Bb A Ab Ab Bb

Colour Sequence: gold - blue - gold - orange - white

Ash *(Fraxinus excelsior)*

Ash is a native forest tree that can grow to 130 feet. The leaves are long and made up of nine to thirteen stalked leaflets that give the tree a light, graceful appearance. Male and female flowers appear before the leaves on the same or on different trees, springing like a gush of water from just behind the black buds at the branch-tips. Ash is usually one of the last trees to come into leaf and the earliest to drop in autumn. The wood is strong, white and flexible – it is said to be able to bear more weight than any other wood. Ash bark has been used as a tonic and astringent, the leaves as a laxative.

Ash brings the strength to stand up for yourself in a way that is in tune with your surroundings. An acknowledgement and exploration of personal status that leads to clear understanding of how one interacts with the world and establishing a harmonious relationship.

The Central meridian, running from the perineum up the front of the body to the lower lip, is strengthened. This stabilises personal energies, vitality and integrity. It ensures the rest of the meridian system is energised.

The root chakra and heart chakra are energised, and this in turn strengthens the sense of reality and the ability to cope with the world, and to feel at home with oneself and the life one is leading.
There is an increase in love and the ability to express feelings in a strong yet compassionate way. There is a steady growth of flexibility and adaptability.

The astral, causal and spiritual subtle bodies are aligned. This balances the Higher Self and its relationship to the collective consciousness, encouraging a sense of security and rightness about one's place in the scheme of things.

Ash was used for the shafts of spears and for bow-making, linking it directly to the Ancestor Wisdom god of the Norse peoples, Odin, Woden, Wode, Wade. Yggdrasil means "horse of Ygg", and Ygg is another name for Odin himself. Odin learnt most of his magical and shamanic powers from earlier chthonic energies.

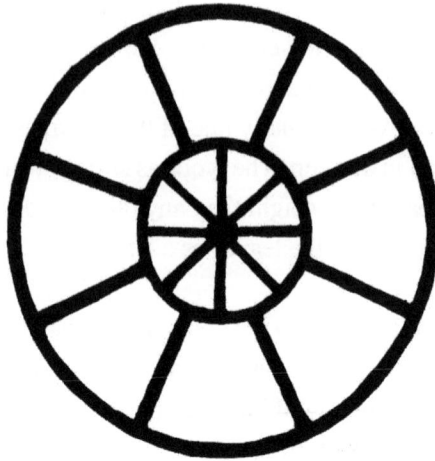

Aspen *(Populus tremula)*

Keyword: delight

Colour: yellow

Chakras: 2, 3

Mantra: CHOO TOE TIE TEA VOO

Note Sequence: D F# D C# Eb Eb C#

Colour Sequence: blue - white - indigo - white - dappled vibrations of light

Aspen *(Populus tremula)*

Aspen is one of the white poplars. It is native to Britain and was one of the pioneer trees to colonise the land when the ice retreated. The aspen is a delicate, open, upright tree that tends to be found in clusters on the edge of woodland in damp soils. Except for the Scottish Highlands it is nowhere widespread, but can be found locally throughout Britain. The tree suckers freely from its shallow roots so many thickets are probably shoots from the same tree. One of the largest organisms on the planet is said to be an aspen in Colorado that covers thousands of acres with genetically identical suckered clones. Aspen has a smooth silvery bark, marked with dark horizontal pores, that darkens and furrows with age. The main energy of aspen is the protection of the soul's wisdom and the ability to manifest wisdom in practical ways.

The Large Intestine meridian can be quite affected by the negative emotional qualities of stuffiness and constipated attitudes, as well as guilt and shame. Aspen brings a sense of humour and an appreciation of one's own failings, which is a great destroyer of fear. Any fear ultimately reduces down to fear of change, fear of letting go.

Aspen has an opening and balancing effect on the mind so that fears are calmed and a space is created within which one can think and organise, reconsidering options for action. The brow chakra is significantly affected. Firstly, there is a soothing and peaceful effect on the over-active imagination. With peace comes the ability to express ideas and concepts that are, by their very nature, difficult to categorize. Intuitive insights and imaginative creativity become a lot easier to share with others in language that can be understood by all.

At the finest spiritual levels aspen again works with the mind, opening and balancing the intellect so that it takes creative potential into its functions. This integrates intuitive insights within the intellect and prevents over-analysis of situations by the rational mind.

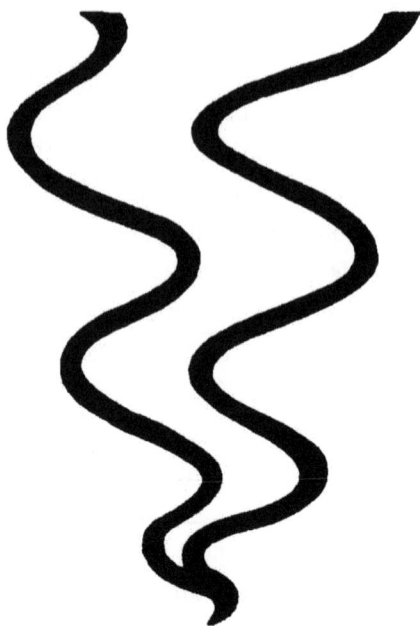

Atlas Cedar *(Cedrus atlantica)*

Keyword: resilience

Colour: green

Chakra: 4

Mantra: YEE OO BAY BAY BAY

Note Sequence: G B G B C# C# B A B

Colour Sequence: Red - green - indigo - gold - red

Atlas Cedar *(Cedrus atlantica)*

Atlas cedar comes from the Atlas Mountains of Algeria and Morocco in North Africa. It has been planted in Britain since 1844 but the largest number of trees are now blue Atlas cedar, a natural variation that is found growing amidst the more common dark green variety in the wild. The tree grows to 35m. (110 ft.) and has slightly ascending, sweeping branches. (The three main cedars planted in Britain can be identified thus : Atlas cedar has Ascending branches, cedar of Lebanon has Level branches, deodar has Descending branches).

The bark of Atlas cedar is a smooth dark grey with fine fissures. Needles grow singly on new growth and in rosettes on mature stems. Like all cedars, the Atlas cedar flowers in autumn. Male flowers are upright, cone-like and pink, turning yellow when heavy with pollen. Small green female flowers become large pot-shaped cones with a sunken top that disintegrates after two years to leave the central spike.

Atlas cedar essence is of great benefit for those who feel they lack a worthwhile direction in their life, or who face opposition to their chosen way of life. It provides the energy to take full advantage of every opportunity and the practical initiative to make something from nothing. Self-confidence increases so there is less need to seek the approval of others.

Atlas cedar helps to clear the etheric body of old, unwanted patterns of energy. These subtle scars can act as focus points for physical problems and reduce the flexibility of the body's systems to deal with new stresses.

There is a greater organisation and flow of information that calms and clarifies deep levels of personal energy patterns. Fears and anxieties are reduced and it becomes easier to see what needs to be done to get the best out of each situation in life. Finally, Atlas cedar brings the ability to experience the underlying creative patterns of the universe. It becomes easier to see the constant flow and change in all things, the continuous re-patterning and re-capitulation of the infinite creative urge without repetition.

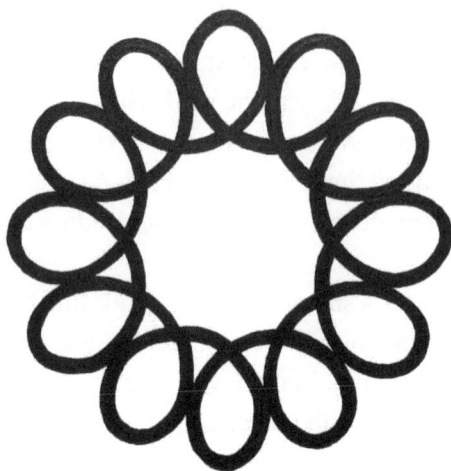

Bay *(Laurus nobilis)*

Keyword: energy

Colour: dark red

Chakra: Earth Star (below the feet)

Mantra: POO RU (x6)

Note sequence: B G

Colour sequence: black - red - black - indigo - violet - green (repeated)

Bay *(Laurus nobilis)*

Bay, sweet bay or bay laurel, is a native of the Mediterranean area. Usually planted in gardens for its aromatic leaves, bay rarely grows higher than twenty-five feet in Britain though it can grow well over twice this height in warmer climates. The entire tree has a high content of aromatic essential oil – the glossy evergreen leaves and smooth, dark purple-brown twigs burn easily with a heavy scented smoke. It is possible that bay smoke was an ingredient of the incense used by Classical oracles, as it is narcotic and excitant. The Oracle of Delphi was the primary religious centre of ancient Greece and was under the protection of the sun god Apollo. Bay laurel was sacred to Apollo. Internally it is a dangerous oil, increasing blood pressure and heart rate. Externally it can be a useful warming poultice for aches and bruises. From Roman times it has had associations with Apollo and protection from harm, both from disease and spiritual harm. The trees are male or female with yellow flowers clustering at the leaf bases in spring. Female trees produce glossy black berries.

Bay essence has a deep-rooted effect on the whole of the body. It gives an energising boost that some may find too strong for comfort. Bay is a deep red energy, strongly grounding, and this may give rise to explosions of energy as blocks are released.

Bay can encourage the expression of suppressed or hidden emotions, particularly strong ones like anger. Combined with apple an effective cleansing of the emotional system can be encouraged.

The tree is very protective. It enhances the entire meridian system and stimulates the physical. At the other end of the spectrum, bay draws down a powerful vortex of spiritual energy through the upper chakras which can remove and neutralise negative thought-forms and other harmful influences.

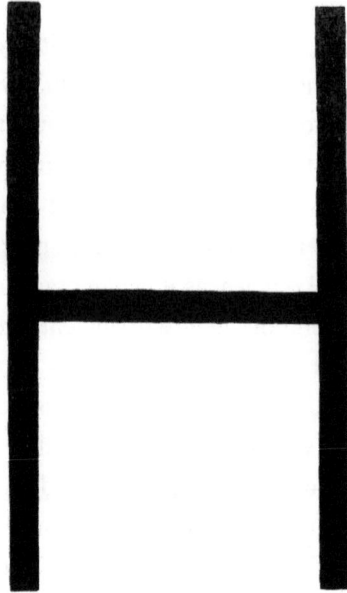

Beech *(Fagus sylvaticus)*

Keyword: easy-going

Colour: orange

Chakra: 2

Mantra: DESH LA CHI

Note sequence: *G *G *F *F D C

Colour sequence: Orange - white - blue - black

Beech *(Fagus sylvaticus)*

Beech will grow easily on any soil except heavy or clay soils (where oak flourishes), and it will eventually come to dominate any woodland, particularly on chalk and limestone uplands. Young trees need to be protected by other species until they are established and are able to tolerate exposed conditions.

Beech has a nearly cylindrical trunk that can reach to 100 feet (30 m) over 120 years. When not crowded beech will start branching fairly close to the ground and these low branches have the characteristic of holding their copper coloured leaves throughout the winter months. The bark is thin, smooth and silver-grey – making beech one of the most beautiful and sensuous looking of trees that grow in Britain.

Beech brings creativity to the highest level of the self. This doesn't necessarily mean any outward form of expression, it is more an internal creativity, a building up of the self within the self – a healing and accepting of one's true nature. This gives confidence and security. There is a relaxation of the area of the solar plexus chakra.

Beech increases hopefulness and confidence. It allows one to release and express personal potential more fully. Fears about the future, despair and loneliness are reduced. Those who lack confidence in speaking, suffer from sore throats, or who have a difficulty in demonstrating their abilities often indicates a block at the throat chakra that beech essence will help to clear.

The emotional body is relaxed where there are difficulties with self-image, particularly in the areas of sexuality and body image. Trauma and shock at the emotional levels can be released, leading to relaxation and a more open, easy-going nature.

At the finer mental levels of the causal body, beech essence brings an easier flow of information and a more harmonious structuring of energy links that results in an increased sense of peacefulness and joy. It also allows a clearer means of expression in a more structured, rational and logical manner.

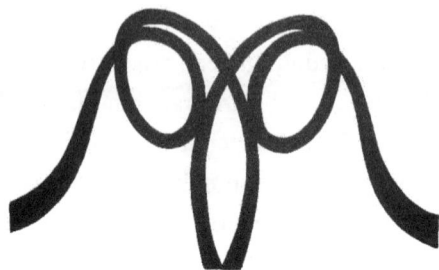

Bird Cherry *(Prunus padus)*

Keyword: sensuality

Colour: pink

Chakra: 4

Mantra: GIY'EE …..GIY'EE

Note Sequence: G D C E G D D C

Colour Sequence: orange - blue - pink

Bird Cherry *(Prunus padus)*

The bird cherry is a smaller native cherry than the gean and is more common in the north of Britain. Varieties are widely planted for their spectacular sprays of white flowers that open in May when the gean has already faded. The fruit is bitter – hence the name, though like many other cherries the bark is useful as a sedative and a tonic infusion

Bird cherry initiates a healing balance and an increase in happiness. There is a noticeable relaxation, particularly of body-awareness and an increased sensuality.

The Gallbladder meridian is cleansed of tension created by a sense of self-righteousness. This increases sense of humour and a more tolerant understanding of the self, one's potential, and acceptance of the possibility for self-healing.

Emotional indifference is eased. There can be deep healing of those emotional wounds, which the outer show of indifference is intended to protect or disguise. Self-criticism and guilt relates to the functions of the Large Intestine meridian and this is energised and balanced with bird cherry. Healing arises when there is a connection of the self to the rest of creation, with the understanding that it is necessary to love and be loved. Feelings of unworthiness, guilt and self-disgust can be dissolved.

The emotional body is freed to enable it to judge more fairly, to see clearly and to communicate true feelings. The mental body can be cleared of negative self-beliefs, increasing the available life-energy and allowing forgiveness.

Signature: The abundant, strongly scented flowers (almond-like, cyanide compounds), displayed in instantly recognisable spikes suggest self- awareness and pleasure in physical existence. An abundance of expression.

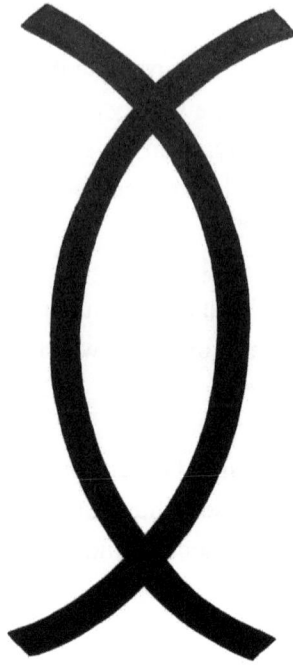

Black Poplar *(Populus nigra)*

Keyword: solidity

Colour: indigo

Chakra: 6

Mantra: J'HAY YAA ROO D'HOO HOO RNAA

Note Sequence: F# D F F# G

Colour Sequence: dark blue - dark red field with gold sparkles - violet

Black Poplar *(Populus nigra)*

Most black poplars in Britain are hybrid varieties planted for rapid growth and effective windbreaks. The true native black poplar is one of the most endangered species in Britain today with only a thousand or so recorded. It can be identified by its birch-like leaves (hybrids have longer and more heart-shaped leaves), and by the rough, heavily burred trunk. Poplars cross-breed easily so exact identification can be difficult. Large male catkins appear in March, a deep red colour. Female trees produce a yellow catkin that elongates to become necklace-like fruit that release large amounts of cotton fine seeds in June. Black poplar is a large spreading tree with thick branches that can reach 100 feet (30 m).

The key for black poplar is solidity and security. It brings about an inner environment where peace can be established as a powerful state. Consciousness is raised to a level of detachment where the reality of situations is recognised from a spiritual, unifying viewpoint. At its finest, this essence brings in universal wisdom and a sense of complete security, at home even in the velvet depths of space.

The brow chakra and throat chakra are stimulated together with the 11th chakra which is located above the head quite some distance from the physical body. This allows fine perceptions and discernment to become integrated with normal behaviour patterns. A link is created between the etheric body and the soul body. This brings spiritual energies closer towards the physical body increasing the sense of confidence and security. The Heart meridian is balanced, increasing the acceptance of love and forgiveness.

Comment: Black poplar is so-named from the deep shadows cast by the knotted, burred and gnarled trunk. The commonly seen Lombardy poplar is an upright, narrow variety of black poplar thought to have originated in Asia and brought to Britain from northern Italy in 1758. The core energy to the native tree is quite similar, as is that of the hybrids, though superficial characteristics tend to modify the expressions of that energy: hybrids have a much lighter, airier feel.

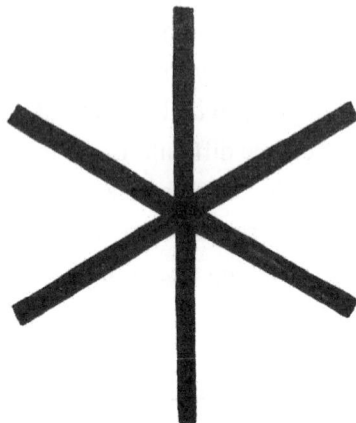

Blackthorn *(Prunus spinosa)*

Keyword: circulation

Colour: red

Chakra: 1

Mantra: JIM OO KO JEE JEE DAY

Note Sequence: C# E F A C# Eb *D (the last D is one octave lower than other notes)

Colour Sequence: yellow - yellow plus pink - violet - white

Blackthorn *(Prunus spinosa)*

Blackthorn is commonly found in hedgerows and at the edge of scrub woodland. Each plant suckers freely to produce dense masses of impenetrable thorn bushes. Blackthorn can become a small tree but never grows much more than 15 feet (4m). It has black, shiny bark with strong sharp spines and a hard orange wood – traditionally the material of cudgels ('shillelagh') because of its heaviness and strength. The densely packed white flowers open in spring before the small leaves appear. (The earliest white blossom in the British countryside is cherry plum, followed by blackthorn, then wild cherry in April, then hawthorn in May.) The fruits, 'sloes', are blue-black and very sour, only becoming fully ripened after the first frosts.

There is a whole-system energising. Hope and joy increases with the lively energising of the Small Intestine meridian and Triple Warmer meridian. The root chakra (survival issues, manifestation, physical skill), and the heart chakra (balancing, integrating, understanding) are positively influenced. A small chakra at the base of the arch of the foot which relates to the functions of the small intestine, is stimulated and this helps the absorption of energy to stabilise emotional states. In these cases other appropriate essences may be one of the maples (silver, field, sycamore). The increase of energy levels helps to counter the effects of sadness, solitude and hopelessness.

Blackthorn is a very protective essence particularly from non-physical entities and other energy patterns that may weaken or infiltrate the subtle spiritual body. There is an overall refinement and integration of fine level energy, a rooting of the spirit into matter.

Signature: The white frosting of blackthorn across the countryside in early spring is sign of returning energy and life to the land. The sharp, spiky thorns emphasise the here-and-now of physical existence. The velvety-purple sloes: spirit growing from the energy of form.
(Simon once saw the spirit of blackthorn as a young warrior girl guided and perhaps guarded by a surly looking, cudgel-wielding dwarf!)

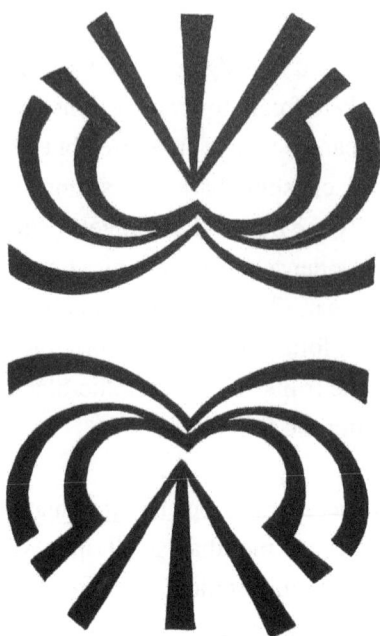

Box Tree *(Buxus sempevirens)*

Keyword: clarity

Colour: white

Chakras: 3,7

Mantra: NYER LERT.   YERRRU   YERRRI

Note Sequence: Ab   C#

Colour Sequence: blue - green - pink - indigo - black

Box Tree *(Buxus sempevirens)*

A few groves of box exist on the chalk and limestone of the North Downs, Chilterns and Cotswolds. Its heavy dense wood is the only native wood that, when green, sinks in water. Being heavily cropped for its timber, few large mature trees now exist in the wild. It can grow to a height of 35 feet (11m). Box has small, dark evergreen leaves and a smooth, finely cracked light brown bark. The yellow flowers appear in April at the leaf axils, each cluster containing up to five male flowers surrounding a central female flower.

Box is a useful essence to stimulate life-energy within the individual. This is particularly appropriate where emotions are involved. Sorrow, disappointment and grief are known to seriously deplete people soon after suffering a significant sadness in their life. Box helps to sustain the flow of positive energy and optimistic view of life.

The Stomach meridian is stimulated and will more effectively cleanse and repair issues of negative self-image, particularly to do with belief systems where there is conflict between desires and feelings of disgust and dirtiness. Understanding and letting go of old conflicts is made possible.

The causal body, connecting self to the collective soul of humanity, is also given healing. There will be an increased feeling of connectedness to the energy of the universe and a reduction of feelings of separation, isolation and unworthiness.

When these false concepts begin to be removed extra energy can be redirected to mental and spiritual states so there is an increase in energy levels and more constructive activity. Strong feelings can now be focused in creative, helpful ways and a greater spiritual maturity can emerge.

Box can also be used as a way to purify and cleanse the atmosphere, both on a physical level as well as from negative or dulling thought-forms and spirit energies.

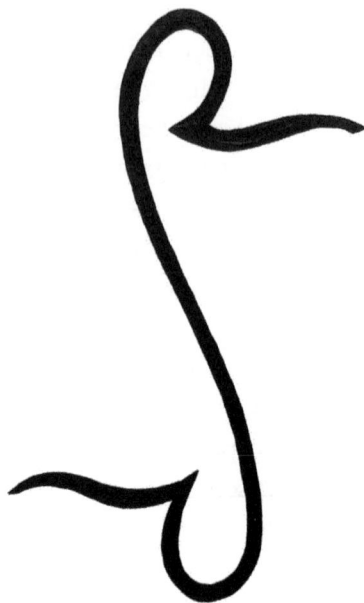

Catalpa (*Catalpa x erubescans)*

Keyword: joy

Colour: yellow

Chakra: 3

Mantra: J'HAY

Note Sequence: G C# C# G

Colour sequence: yellow ochre - red ochre - dark brown

Catalpa *(Catalpa x erubescans)*

The catalpa, also called the Indian bean tree, is named from the native American tribe, the Catawba of the Louisiana and Florida regions. Catalpas are sensitive to frost so they are usually only found in the south of Britain. It comes into leaf very late in June, and it flowers in August or September. Flowers appear on large spikes, somewhat similar to horse chestnut 'candles', but more open. The flowers of the hybrid catalpa, a cross between the southern catalpa from America and the yellow catalpa from China, was introduced into Britain in 1891 and has a sweet, powerful scent. In winter the tree is characterised by its long, bean-like seed pods, in summer by its huge leaves.

The quality of catalpa is primarily in the increase of peace and the calming of anxieties. There is a stabilisation of the emotions.

The Small Intestine meridian is supported. This is the channel that becomes stressed by sadness and sorrow, and energised by joy and happiness. There is a general calming of the emotions and of the energy pulses at various parts of the body. Very often these pulses can be felt to be out of synchrony when a person is under stress, falling back into rhythm as the stress is lifted. Catalpa essence placed on these pulse points (like the wrists, the frontal eminences on the forehead and the tops of the little fingers), would help to regulate these subtle energies very quickly.

As the body calms down the mind can achieve a new state of balance and discrimination. The energies of this tree are largely focused on balancing the polarity of the intuition and the intellect, the personal wants with the appropriate needs, the flow of personal expression and will, and the balance of happiness and fear.

The lifting of conflicts, both emotional and mental, can lead to a greater sense of security and connectedness into the surroundings and even an increased ability to use psychic and other skills in a useful way.

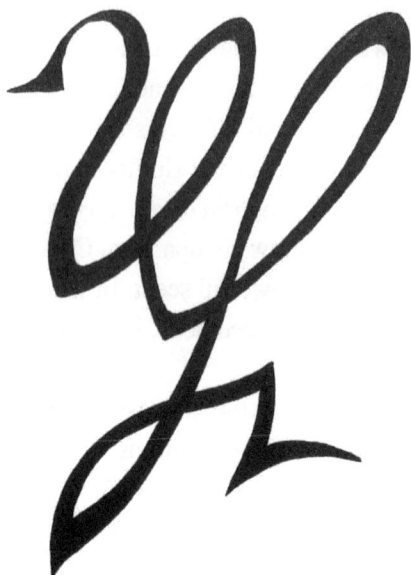

Cedar of Lebanon *(Cedrus libani)*

Keyword: turmoil

Colour: green

Chakra: 4

Mantra: TUSS EYE TUH GHEE SIGH

Note Sequence: * A *E G A B G* E*
(asterisks denote lower octaves if before the note, upper octaves if after the note)

Colour Sequence: orange - green - blue

Cedar of Lebanon *(Cedrus libani)*

This familiar parkland tree is characterised by its dark green foliage arranged in flat planes on horizontal branches. Male flowers release pollen in autumn fertilising small female flowers that become barrel-shaped cones. This cedar, with strong, durable, aromatic wood was used so much in ancient shipbuilding and temple construction that the huge forests of the Levant were destroyed leaving the arid, desert conditions of today. It was introduced into Britain in 1636.

There is, overall, a quietening of emotional turmoil. A reduction in mental and emotional friction encourages a deep peacefulness that can reveal one's own foundation of peace.

When there is confusion and despair this essence brings a wordless understanding. There is relaxation, acceptance and a lessening of any resistance to necessary change. With this letting go there is the ability to hear clearer messages from the deep mind and the universe regarding appropriate actions.

Signature: The visual stability and sense of balance: strong-branched, level-headed. The aromatic scent is warm, relaxing and preserving.

Physically cleansing, a breath of fresh air. Where there is suffering this essence lessens the resistance to needed change.

Clearer messages from the deep mind and universe regarding appropriate actions. Increases peaceful flow and reduces turmoil.

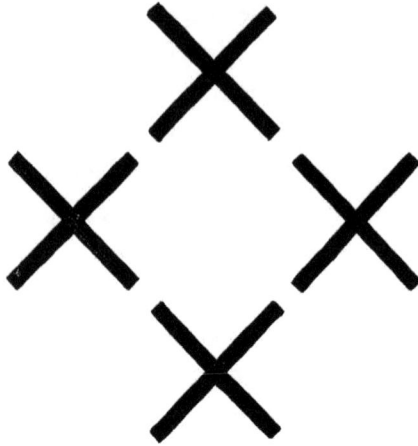

Cherry Laurel *(Prunus laurocerasus)*

Keywords: balance of mind

Colour: violet

Chakra: 7

Mantra: SHOE INGOO HOO. ING (uh) ING (ih)

Note Sequence: F# *G Bb* C# *F#

Colour Sequence: blue - indigo - orange - pink with yellow sparkles

Cherry Laurel *(Prunus laurocerasus)*

This is the well-known laurel planted as a hedging plant for which it has been used since its introduction into Britain in 1576. It is, in fact, a bird cherry of the *Prunus* family originating from around the Caspian and Black Sea. In the past its major use was in creating a dense ground and woodland cover for game birds. Tolerant of shade and moisture it can be very invasive and its shiny evergreen foliage can reach up to 20ft (6m) – though it can be quite startling to see cherry laurel as a tree in its own right, rather than a clipped hedge. The flower spikes are visible early in spring around April, giving off a heady sweet scent from the creamy yellow flowers. Like all cherries this laurel contains a high proportion of prussic acid and when the leaves are crushed they give off the distinctive almond scent of hydrocyanic acid. The flowers ripen to shiny black berries eaten by birds.

The essence focuses on bringing balance to the mental. It will quickly release shock, even from near-death experiences. Cherry laurel allows imagination to be used in a constructive way, enabling more of one's personal potential to be expressed. Imagination and inspiration is greatly enhanced.

The brow chakra is energised in a way that quietens mental activity to such a degree that a depth and clarity of subtle perceptions and insights are able to be identified. This can help with all forms of spiritual communication and channelling. This is also aided by the activation of the crown chakra where the finest levels of the self are linked more closely to the underlying universal sources. This allows an influx of universal harmony, connectedness and fine spiritual energy into the self. The energy link is inherently protective, non-aggressive and supportive, and in this way all aspects of the mind can be made whole, holistic and healed.

It is easy to ignore the trees that have become associated with the domestic and suburban environments, but these are the ones to which many people have the most familiar links – albeit mostly unconscious. It is all too common for these trees to be despised as 'introductions', non-natives, weeds, as though they are of lesser value than other species.

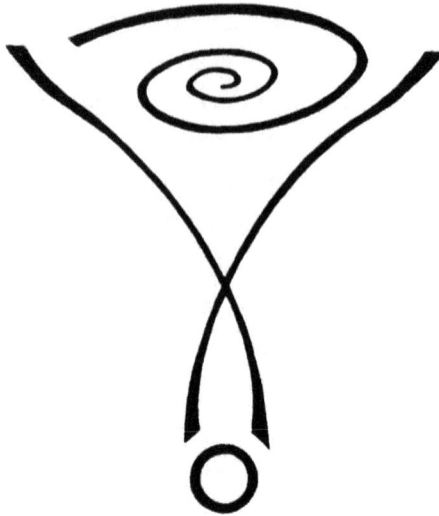

Cherry Plum *(Prunus cerasifera)*

Keyword: confidence

Colours: orange, blue

Chakra: 5

Mantra: VRR... DUH DRR... KEH LUH

Note Sequence: *G *A *F *C# *C *C#

Colour Sequence: orange - white

Cherry Plum *(Prunus cerasifera)*

Also called the myrobalan plum, it is a semi-wild little tree originally from eastern Europe and Central Asia. It is the earliest white blossom to appear in the hedgerows and can be distinguished from blackthorn as the flowers are usually more sparse and delicate with a touch of green from the young leaf-shoots. Cherry plum flowers in February or early March and can grow to be an open-crowned spreading tree of 25 ft. (7.5 m). A purple-leaved variety, *Pissardii*, is commonly planted in gardens. This is a natural sport that arose in the Shah of Persia's gardens in the late 19th century and was sent to France. It has pinkish flowers.

The essence of cherry plum helps to remove fears and anxiety by uncovering the wisdom and ultimate security of the inner self. Tensions that are locked into the muscle system relating to such fears and mental attitude can be eased. The Central meridian (Conception Vessel) strengthens to improve self-confidence. This combats shyness and brings about a space to develop a fuller personal potential.

The throat chakra is energised and enabled to make practical use of subtle perceptions, intuition, inspiration and so on. Communication and artistic blocks are eased. At the same time the crown chakra becomes clearer allowing more healing, universal energies to merge and harmonise with the localised identity of the self at a safe rate and pace. The sense of time and space is relaxed so that the present comes into better focus and can be honestly experienced as it is.

As well as this connection with stabilising universal energies cherry plum also allows a better connection with others at an emotional, feeling level. This helps to balance the emotions and suggests that cherry plum would be useful for those who are affected by strong emotional swings.

Mentally this tree essence brings a deep peace and serenity, quietening the heart and mind and allowing the inner self to come through.

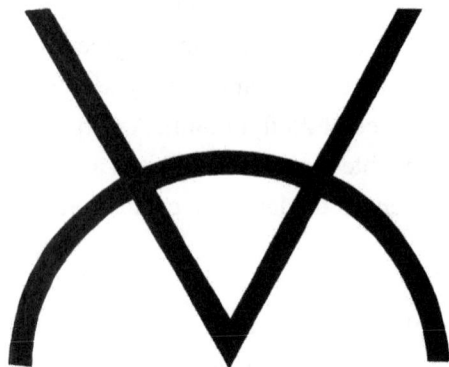

Copper Beech *(Fagus sylvatica var. purpurea)*

Keyword: depression

Colours: blue, gold, magenta

Chakras: 2, 6

Mantra: DOO VAA TEA... TEA BUY D'HEE

Note Sequence: E F D E G

Colour Sequence: brown - orange - play of dark rainbow tones

Copper Beech *(Fagus sylvatica var. purpurea)*

Copper beech was first recorded as growing in Switzerland in 1680 and later also arose at least a couple of times in Germany. Its form and habit is identical to the common green variety except that its foliage is a deep reddish-purple colour. Copper beech is mainly found as a garden or park tree where its colour stands out dramatically amongst the surrounding vegetation.

The emotions are energised, but in a positive way. Anger and repressed, or otherwise inappropriate, emotions are expelled in a non-aggressive, positive way. There is a greater understanding and acceptance of the individual's deep unconscious emotional tendencies and instincts – the patterns of behaviour that automatically trigger in certain situations. Emotional difficulties with relationships are eased. Copper beech helps to see each situation as it is, rather than being viewed through a distorting screen of past experience.

There is the possibility to relieve depressive thoughts and bring a deep, enlivening sense of peace and detachment from worries as stress is lifted from these aspects of the Lung meridian. The emotional body becomes better balanced giving a sense of easiness and humour. There is a more relaxed ability to accept and express lovingly who one is and what one feels.

There is a greater positive receptivity; an ability to be peaceful without a need to do something else. It can be useful in depression or when there is need of greater emotional independence or detachment from an emotional situation.

At extremely fine, universal levels this tree helps to sharpen intelligence, clarity and the sense of joy.

Signature: The purple-red leaves appear sombre and weighty yet allow a red light to filter through. This feels quietening and energising. Magenta, pink and red are the qualities of this essence together with an indigo-purple.

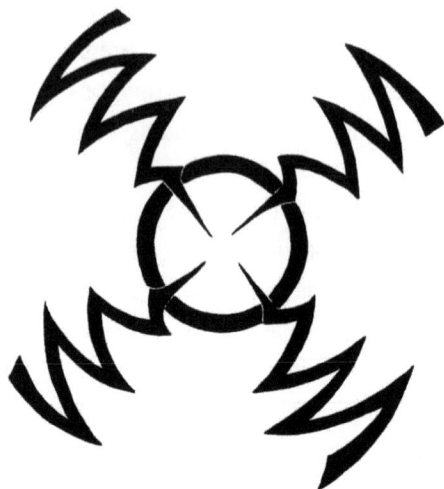

Crack Willow *(Salix fragilis)*

Keywords: spiritual sun

Colour: yellow

Chakra: 3

Mantra: PL OO. G'DHOO. JI - NOW

Note sequence: Ab C Ab Db A Eb

Colour sequence: violet - indigo - yellow - turquoise

Crack Willow *(Salix fragilis)*

Just about a quarter of the native species of British trees are willows. Whether native or introduced, all species interbreed freely often making precise identification difficult. Crack willow is one of the largest species growing to between 30 and 40 ft. It has a wide, open crown, often with several trunks spreading outwards from the base, and a rough, thick-ridged bark. It can be identified from its leaves which are long, thin blades with fine serrated edges ending in a long point. When touched or bent this willow's small twigs will easily break with an audible crack – hence the tree's name. This quality allows twigs to float downstream where they can easily root in mud and form new colonies.

Crack willow essence increases communication with the Higher Self, often by stimulating the functions of the throat chakra. It can be used to stimulate and awaken physical vitality as it begins to wane throughout the day. There is an increased flexibility on mental and spiritual levels. This allows the individual to be content to let things be, for things to happen in their own good time, to let go. With this comes the ability to look at oneself and accept what is seen.

A connection is created with compassionate energies at fine levels of consciousness, and this brings a sense of oneness with the world and all beings in it. Also there is created a stronger link to the planet itself, and through this, to the place from which Earth receives its sustaining energies – that is, the sun. Crack willow particularly links to the higher vibrations of the sun's energies that have been personified as the Solar Logos, which is, as it were, the parent and creator of the whole solar system.

Signature: The ability to let go of parts of oneself (the twigs) in the knowledge that they will find a home elsewhere.

Comment: Willows are often associated with water, the moon and the dark aspects of the Goddess but they carry just as many solar characteristics as lunar aspects.

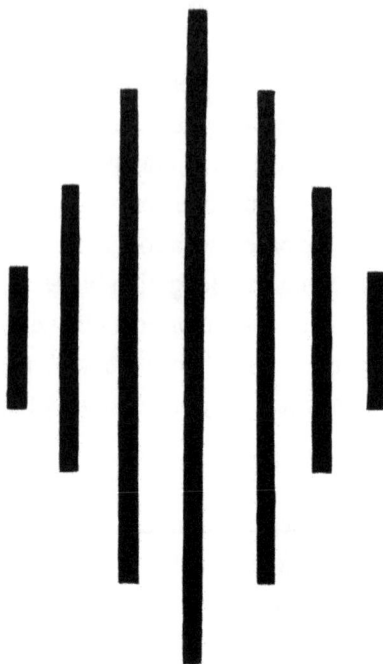

Douglas Fir *(Pseudotsuga menziesii)*

Keywords: standing alone

Colour: green

Chakra: 4

Mantra: SAY GEE B' HAA TOO GEE B'HAA HRRR(uh)

Note Sequence: Ab G D D Eb D

Colour Sequence: blue - yellow - flashing black/white - gold (repeated sequence)

Douglas Fir *(Pseudotsuga menziesii)*

Douglas fir is a magnificent tree, one of the largest in the world. It is native to North America and makes up a significant proportion of the temperate rainforest of the Pacific North-West coast.

Douglas fir is named after David Douglas who sent seed to the Horticultural Society in 1827. The Latin name remembers Archibald Menzies who first found the tree and sent a sample of foliage to Kew Gardens in 1793. Douglas fir has a corded, corky bark of dark grey or purple. Its foliage is held on large down-swept branches and is a dense covering of rich dark green that deeply shades the ground underneath. The leaves have a sweet, fruity scent. Cones can be identified by the papery 'tongues' that emerge between the scales.

The primary energy of Douglas fir concerns itself with finding space to be and to act as oneself. All aspects of this relationship with the world outside, and to finding one's place in the world, are brought into a better balance with this tree's help. It gives the dynamism for spontaneous activity, which is nonetheless appropriate and balanced. Energy to grow and space to act are easier to find.

The Triple Warmer meridian is concerned with the maintenance of the body's own internal systems, ensuring a correct working relationship between organs. When imbalance is found in this meridian Douglas fir will naturally help to restore calm equilibrium. Where there is a need to feel part of a group, of belonging and being valued, as serving a useful function in a group but where there is also a need to be apart from the pressures and commitments of complex relationships, this tree essence will help to resolve the opposing tensions.

At the most refined level Douglas fir brings us the clarity of awareness to recognise this connection between all individual selves. It helps to cleanse and purify those separating and limiting belief patterns that prevent the true expansion of self-awareness. Ultimately helping to realise a sense of self, of unique being-ness, of existence.

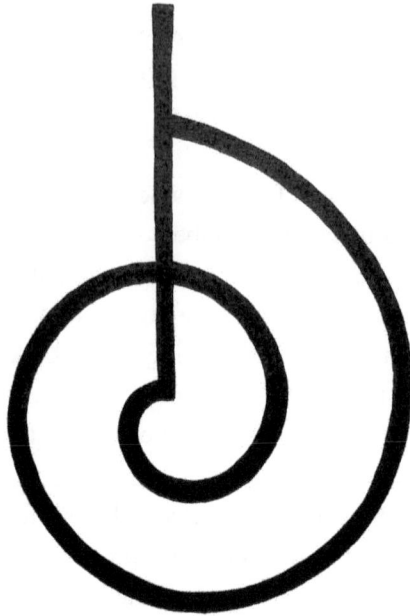

Elder *(Sambucus nigra)*

Keywords: self-worth

Colour: pink

Chakra: 4

Mantra: MOO GUS GAAAD

Note sequence: *E *G *B *F *F
 (prefix * shows notes in octave below Middle C)

Colour sequence: blue - gold - pale pink

English Elm *(Ulmus procera)*

There are many varieties of elm with very similar forms. The English elm was characterised by its tall, narrow crown with dense foliage growing close to the boughs. It could reach a height of 120 ft. (36m). All elms, except wych elm, sucker freely and even with the continuing ravages of Dutch elm disease hedgerows still contain many young elms, easily identified by their vigorous branches at a regular angle of about 45 degrees to the main trunk and the clearly alternate large leaves. The flowers are small and appear on the twigs early in the year well before the leaves appear, giving the whole tree a reddish tinge.

The essence of elm brings the ability to organise fine levels of information or energy in a way that can be easily understood. It allows a greater ability to have an overview of any situation, giving discrimination and sufficient detachment. There is also the possibility of knowledge from the beyond.

The Large Intestine meridian is also affected with an increased ability to cleanse and remove foreign materials by establishing correct sense of personal boundaries, increased sense of purpose and direction. Clarification of who one is allows identification of what one wishes to distance oneself from.

Elm brings the ability to experience and understand others on a level of feeling. Emotions are stabilised. There is an increase in equilibrium and compassion and the ability to give and receive love. It also becomes possible to determine more accurately the validity of personal actions, balancing the qualities of conscience and guilt feelings. Many chakras around the heart and abdomen are brought into balance. The brow chakra, too, is boosted creating a dynamic calm that allows experience of fine perception and transcendence of normal states of consciousness.

Confusion, oppression and fatigue are reduced making decisions easier. Elm is a useful essence to use to re-energise the mind when fatigued and balance the heart chakra when feeling drained or over-emotional.

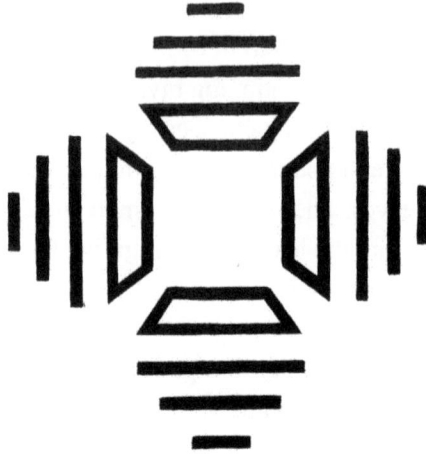

Eucalyptus (Cider Gum) *(Eucalyptus gunnii)*

Keyword: sustenance

Colour: green

Chakra: 4

Mantra: CH' RRR(uh) KOO G' HAY

Note Sequence: G A *G *F *E *G *Ab *F *Ab *Ab

Colour Sequence: orange - green

Eucalyptus (Cider Gum) *(Eucalyptus gunnii)*

The Eucalyptus family is native to Australia and Tasmania. It contains over three hundred species, which are adapted to conditions of heat and dryness by having leaves that are thick and leathery and that turn their edges towards the sun to reduce evaporation.

Eucalyptus creates the space we need to be creative, and also brings the discipline needed to creatively organise our energies. It becomes easier to take advantage of the existing conditions in a way that benefits our lives. Intuition, our grasp of larger patterns and underlying energy fluctuations, is brought into a better relationship with the feelings of the body. With this intuitive body wisdom, awareness becomes more firmly rooted in the senses and the body, helping us feel more in control of our lives, calm and integrated.

A dynamic energy is set up in the Central meridian, balancing the life energy there. Eucalyptus will help to direct the individual to those types of practical activity that help to maintain the integrity of this important energy channel. It will encourage whatever is required to grow and become more powerful in oneself.

All the chakras are helped by the energy of eucalyptus to have a more efficient, interactive functioning. It brings an increase in energy and a better distribution of resources, so that the whole body works more smoothly and is better able to cope with new stress and more effective at releasing existing stresses in the body. A quality of space and freedom is also felt in the mind. It becomes easier to see things more clearly and in original ways. Eucalyptus brings a discipline to organise and to make the most of any situation because it can help to reveal the most important underlying truths.

At subtle levels eucalyptus takes the mind to the very finest levels of awareness. This makes it a useful essence for mantra meditation and those types of contemplative practice that involve witnessing.

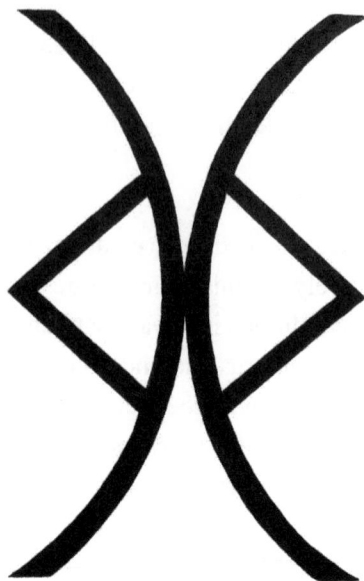

Field Maple *(Acer campestre)*

Keywords: aching heart

Colour: pink

Chakra: 4

Mantra: TRRRIH VOO HRRRUH VAY

Note Sequence: F# Eb F#

Colour Sequence : brick red - indigo - white

Field Maple *(Acer campestre)*

Field maple is the only species of this family native to Britain. It is quite common on chalky soils but is often not very obvious though it can grow to a tree up to 85 feet (26 metres). The leaves have the familiar maple shape but are simpler with three main rounded lobes. The leaves unfold a pink colour and become a butter yellow in autumn. The small upright clusters of flowers in spring are green and not very noticeable. The clearest time to identify field maple in the hedgerows is around the summer solstice when a second growth shows a bright red. The burring and knots on the main trunk made field maple a decorative wood until replaced by imported maple woods.

There can be total security within the self that allows unconditional love to be given and received. Field maple acts as a balance to those who desperately seek love without looking inside themselves to discover what may be pushing that love away. Once achieved inside, love will appear wherever one looks. This essence draws down a high wisdom energy from above the crown chakra and helps to establish it in the solar plexus chakra where it is able to manifest its power.

There is understanding and a contentment for those who are overwhelmed by remorse or a sense of being responsible for events and accidents. It can rebalance after shock. Field maple enables one to return to centre.

It opens and balances the heart chakra allowing an expansion of the awareness of relationships to others and being part of an integrated universal web of interaction and growth. The consciousness of universal love.

Emotional problems are calmed, especially where there is anger or over-aggression. This is because field maple balances the love aspects of the self. At the finest levels of energy this tree establishes a fine limited from the absolute, indefinable levels of creation, the void, to that place where boundaries and the relative levels of existence begin to emerge.When this region becomes familiar it links one to an infinite source of awareness and power where self and universe merge.

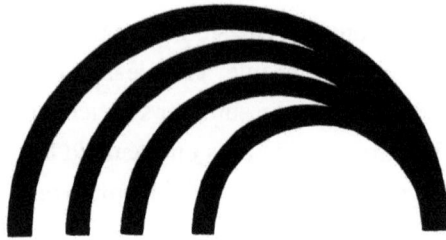

Fig Tree *(Ficus carica)*

Keyword: generator

Colours: red, orange

Chakra: 1

Mantra: VRRRUH VRRRIH VO VOW

Note Sequence: F E C *D *D *F *C

Colour Sequence: darkness - red - orange - green - darkness

Fig Tree *(Ficus carica)*

The earliest record of figs in Britain is from the beginning of the 16th century, though there are references to much earlier plantings, and certainly the Romans may have established figs in their farm villas. The leaves are easily recognisable with thick, leathery, hairy surfaces with between three to five deep rounded lobes. The flower of the fig is completely inside the immature fruit and is pollinated only by a small gall wasp that burrows its way through the skin. Figs fruit twice a year: in May the fruits ripen in the warm weather but these are often destroyed by the cold of the autumn months. Edible figs tend to be those that bud later in the year and survive the winter to swell in the following spring and summer.

The fig tree has a tightly defined sphere of action: it echoes the moment of creation where a single burst of energy manifested the universe. It contains the compassionate energy of life and the awareness of dynamic love. It holds the understanding that all things exist as part of one single creative impulse, fragments of a single creativity bomb. Fig tree helps to energise areas of stagnancy and coolness, where the natural flow of energy has ceased to move in a normal way. The cause of static energy could be the failure to express honesty – the inability or reluctance of the individual to maintain and uphold their own energy integrity, their own right to exist as a unique entity.

The Governor meridian along the spinal column will be given a boost of energy that may release pent-up and unexpressed feelings and ideas. With this there will also arise a clearer message to others of your personal need for space and freedom. Fig tree will turn the attention back to the causes of discomfort within oneself and help to resolve it there where it started, instead of continually mirroring dissatisfaction outwards onto the world.

The mind is helped to become calm and creative, allowing one to see what is needed to flow into harmonious living again. At spiritual levels, too, fears are calmed and clarity increases. It becomes easier to communicate ideas and information, to access far memory – memory from deep parts of oneself or from the akashic records of creation .

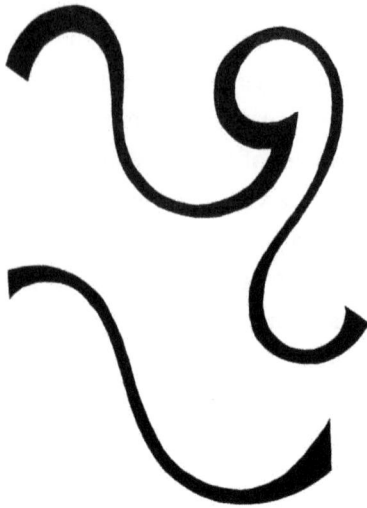

Foxglove Tree *(Pawlownia tomentosa)*

Keywords: harmonious flow

Colour: indigo

Chakra: 6

Mantra: GAA CHAI GAA GHAI CHAI

Note Sequence: E C C C C C F D D

Colour Sequence: indigo

Foxglove Tree *(Pawlownia tomentosa)*

The Latin name of the foxglove tree derives from the daughter of Tsar Paul I of Russia, Anna Paulownia, who became the wife of King William II. The tree was first discovered by Westerners in Japan by a German botanist, E. Kaemfer, in the 17th century. It is native to China where it has been highly regarded as a bringer of health and longevity.

Foxglove tree has a powerful action on the underlying and fundamental energies of the body. It has the ability to help in the removal of emotional blocks – caused by emotional wounds, shocks and traumas. Foxglove tree energy can be of great use in quietening a turbulent mind. Like those who continually have radio or television playing in the background suddenly feel uncomfortable when there is no noise, so the mind can feel unnerved when there is a reduction of background thought and it immediately 'turns up the volume' to familiar levels. Foxglove tree makes it easy to accept new levels of quietness in the mind – caused mainly through an increase in efficiency that has resulted from the reduction of turbulence and stress. In a noisy mind, silence is often equated with emptiness and a loss of individual identity. Here, silence is now experienced as a natural function of the easy flow of energy and so causes little concern.

A similar state of flow and intuitive understanding occurs within the emotions, which also naturally reduce their activity to levels appropriate to the time and place. Emotional states arise and are expressed in a natural, easy way. They are neither held onto beyond the time they are relevant, nor are they suppressed because of a belief that they might be wrong in some way. The ease and flow that this essence brings to the whole system ensures that a genuine expression of the individuality is maintained without creating turbulence or upset to those around.

At its finest level foxglove tree takes the harmonious flow of the individual energy patterns and integrates them within a transpersonal, universal pattern. Support, integration and an ability to transcend personal limitations, however those may be conceived, is possible at this level.

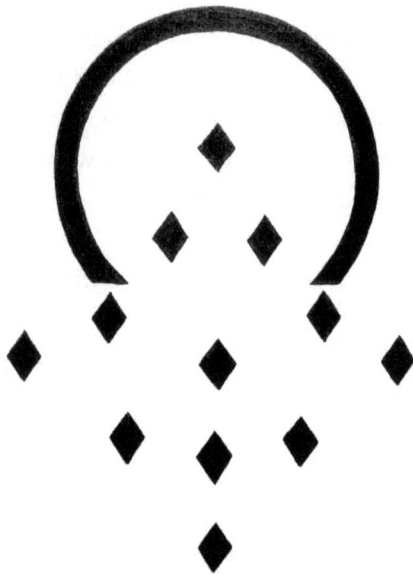

Gean (Wild Cherry) *(Prunus avium)*

Keyword: soothing.

Colour: pink

Chakras: 1, 2, 4

Mantra: CHO PAA T. R. PAA (CHO to rhyme with 'blow')

Note sequence: D D G A B G E C *A

Colour sequence: Turquoise - gold - turquoise - pink

Gean (Wild Cherry) *(Prunus avium)*

The gean or mazzard is a native British cherry of woodlands that grows to 80 feet (25m). In April and May clusters of white flowers emerge from chubby terminal buds before the leaves are fully out. Gean is the original stock from which domestic cherries derive, though most of the wild fruit is taken by animals and birds. The bark is characteristically shiny red-brown with horizontal banding. Cherry wood is compact, fine-grained and heavy. All green parts of the tree have a high content of hyocyanic acid that helps protect from predation.

Gean helps one to let go of unwanted patterns of behaviour, particularly where there is a problem with self-image such as during times of illness. This essence will help with transitions of all kinds.

Sacral chakra and solar plexus chakra are released from stress, again focusing where there are damaging or negative self-beliefs to do with sensuality, sexuality, creativity and physicality.

Gean has a soothing effect. Energy tends to be focused into the physical system and thus stimulate self-healing. This energy flow enters smoothly into the subtle nervous system and helps to balance the whole system. As the channels are cleared the sensation of pain is naturally reduced (pain is the body's indication of a concentration or block of flow).

With gean it is possible to begin the process of purification and cleansing that allows growth and change into life. There can be a new clarity that arises from a greater understanding of self-compassion and acceptance. With this calm and clarity there can be an increase of psychic skills including the perception of subtle beings and gaining access to ancient wisdom.

Comment: wild cherry tree spirit can be one of the most useful energies from which to ask aid wherever there is fear caused by disease or illness. The spirit re-establishes a caring, life-supporting contact with the physical which is often denied such support by the fearful mind.

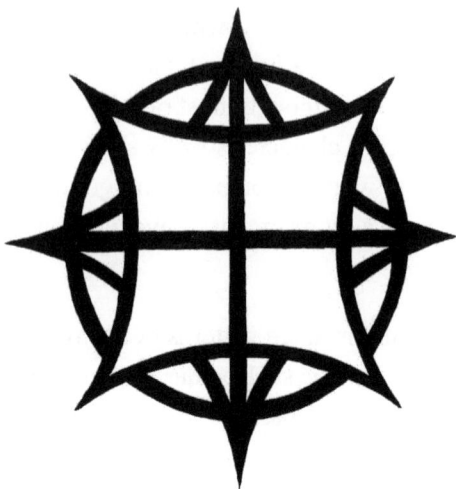

Giant Redwood *(Sequoiadedron giganteum)*

Keywords: weight of responsibility

Colour: green

Chakra: 4

Mantra: NAA FAA KOO SHI

Note sequence: *B F# Eb F# G C#

Colour sequence: green - gold - violet - red

Giant Redwood *(Sequoiadedron giganteum)*

This tree, native only to the inland slopes of the Sierra Nevada mountain range in central California, is the largest tree in the world. The circumference of the base of the trunk can reach 200ft. Younger trees have characteristic downswept branches that are usually shed in mature trees of well over 3,000 years old. It has a deep green, rounded crown of scaly, sharp-pointed leaves growing to 250 ft. Flowers are small cone-like developments on branch endings.
Discovered in 1853, the first seeds were sent to Britain in 1853, the year the Duke of Wellington died. Disease resistant and wind-firm, it quickly became a feature of estates and gardens.

The Bladder meridian is brought to a better balance helpful to identify direction in life; the Lung meridian is helped to increase tolerance; the Gall Bladder to increase the sense of love and forgiveness. It thus helps those who can be too hard on themselves and on others.

Activity is focused at the sacral and throat chakras. Relaxation that allows energy to flow and clear decisions to be made. An increase of flexibility in methods of communication and a greater moderation and appreciation of personal desires, both in oneself and others.

There is a greater chance of balancing human and spiritual values, and of balancing relationship of self to the outside world. Whether this concerns over-involvement with others or an inability to share giant redwood will achieve a workable balance that reduces the stress of such situations.

The mental body is cleared of blocks to creativity and to understanding. Fixed, outmoded belief systems, which tend to create frozen or fixed muscle tension, are eased and so the muscles are helped to relax.

Signature: The ability of older trees to lose unnecessary weight by shedding lower branches.

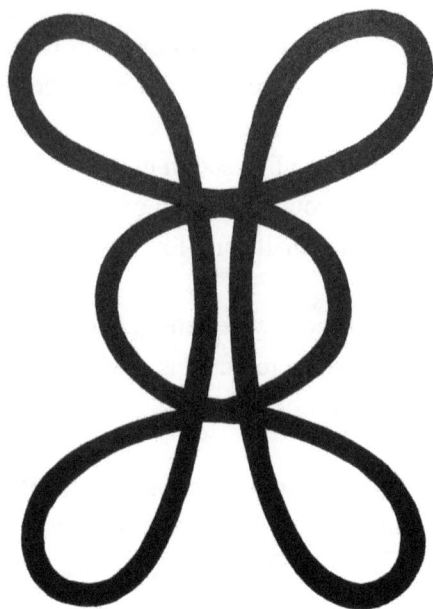

Ginkgo *(Ginkgo biloba)*

Keywords: the ancient way

Colour: indigo

Chakras: 2, 5

Mantra: TIE RNUH BHAA

Note Sequence: G E C D F E D E D

Colour Sequence: white...

Ginkgo *(Ginkgo biloba)*

The ginkgo, or maidenhair tree, is perhaps the most ancient of trees still in existence. It is the only species in its family and has been found as fossilised remains that are over 180 million years old throughout the world. Although it is deciduous, ginkgo is usually classed as a conifer, but in fact it is even older than the conifers, that are considered to be the earliest of the flowering trees.

The main energy of ginkgo helps the internal flow of the feelings within the individual. Ginkgo brings a deep relaxation, a release of emotional stress that allows us to enjoy simple pleasures.

The solar plexus chakra is balanced at emotional and mental levels. Welling up of strong feelings like anger, fear and resentment are quickly brought to a state of peace. That energy is given creative pathways to revivify the life energy in the body, rather than dissipating in emotional outbursts. With this internal harmonisation of flow it becomes possible feel the flow of energy between yourself and others. This can help to balance those who find that they are overly sensitive to the energy of others or who feel they need to be isolated and cut off from the unbalancing influence of other people.

Very deep stresses are helped to clear from the most subtle layers of the body. Tendencies from other lives or from ancestral and genetic patterns begin to work free and lose their hold on behaviour and belief structures. Traumas that have locked the body into working in a certain way are gently melted so that a more creative, stress-free flow of energy can be established.

With this tree's energy comes a profound cleansing and purifying that ultimately can link the flow of the individual's personal energy circuits to the energy circuits of the Universal tides, in harmony of the Universe. In this sense ginkgo creates a state of invisibility. The individual creates no ripples, leaves no footprints, has no power except the perfect amount required to complete each task.

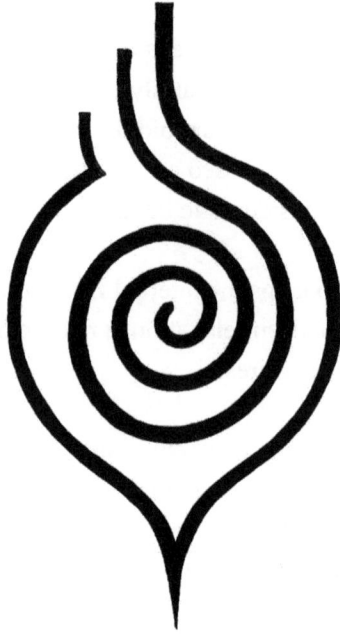

Glastonbury Thorn *(Crataegus monogyna biflora)*

Keywords: out of the woods

Colour: green

Chakra: 4

Mantra: SH' TOO ING INGUH MAA VOO

Note Sequence: Eb D F Eb C D F D

Colour Sequence: white - violet - black and white - violet - black

Gorse *(Ulex europeus, Ulex gallica)*

Gorse rarely becomes large enough to be called a tree. It can grow to 7ft. (2m) even in its usual habitat of windswept heathland. The sharp spines that cover the flexible branches are in fact the plant's evergreen leaves. The coconut-scented flowers open in golden yellow profusion around the end of April, though gorse flowers can be seen throughout the year. There are several different species of gorse showing slight variations of form and time of flowering.

The main characteristic of gorse is the integration of heart and mind. This enables a synthesis of many different ideas and re-energises old, established or forgotten patterns of information in a way that proves useful to the individual outlook.

These new forms of energy/information become better integrated into the physical energy patterns from the much finer subtle bodies from which they emerge. This ensures that they are much more likely to be of practical value. As a result there is an increase in joy arising from a greater feeling of security and growth.

Gorse brings fine levels of positive energy from subtle, universal levels and fully integrates them within the emotional and feeling bodies so that they can be easily expressed in activity.

The meridians of the Bladder and Circulation-Sex (Pericardium) are strengthened. This eases restlessness, frustration and jealousy - states arising from discomfort with the individual's own situation and the seeming inability to change that situation. Some smaller chakras within the lower abdomen are also given energy, enhancing creativity, joy, inner stability, power, healing potential and balanced sexuality.

Dr Edward Bach used gorse for those experiencing hopelessness and despair, convinced that no improvement would be possible. The golden flowers bringing energy and hope of the bright sunlight into people's hearts again.

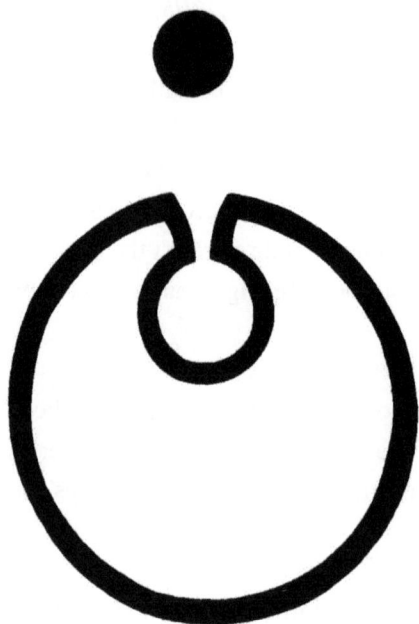

Great Sallow *(Salix caprea)*

Keyword: soul

Colour: yellow

Chakra: 3

Mantra: SHOO GRUHUH ROO DAA

Note sequence: *G Bb Db Bb C (x3)

Colour sequence: gold - red

Great Sallow (*Salix caprea*)

Great sallow, also known as goat willow, is a small, many-stemmed tree that can grow to 50 ft. (15m). It is the well-known 'pussy-willow' with silky, silver buds on the female plants in early spring. Like all willows, male and female flowers appear on separate trees. Great sallow is one of the earliest willows to flower in early spring. The male flowers are grey becoming yellow when fully ripe with pollen, the female flowers are greenish white. A very common tree in Britain, great sallow colonises waste ground, especially damp places, woodlands, scrub and hedgerows. It will also spread onto drier soils.

Great sallow, like others of the willow family, is an energiser. It works to stimulate and motivate the mind in practical, dynamic ways. Both the solar plexus chakra and the eighth chakra located above the head are activated, and this creates a link with the soul through which the conscious awareness can expand. The result is a greater understanding of life purpose that leads to a release of tension. This in turn allows a greater energising of the whole body. Rigidity in the area of the knees can ease which creates a better link to earth energy.

The other major influence of this essence is to bring a profound calm and balance into the whole system. The heart chakra and Heart meridian are stimulated for greater understanding of others, and the relationship of self to others. There is a greater appreciation of the needs of others and a balanced acceptance of personal responsibility and willingness to help, without compromising personal space. Great sallow will help those who are either too involved or those who avoid relationships.

All the different aspects of the subtle self are brought into a greater harmony, and this particularly helps to remove self-defeating behaviour patterns.

The mind, the whole conscious levels of awareness and the higher spiritual energies are brought to a place of calmness and balance from which personal power and steady growth can evolve.

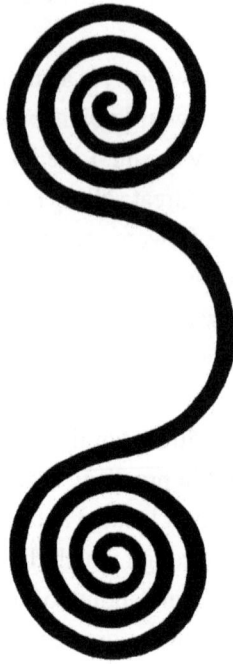

Hawthorn *(Crataegus monogyna)*

Keyword: love

Colours: pink, green

Chakra: 4

Mantra: MAA ILCH DUH HUH RRR FIY

Note sequence: D B D D

Colour sequence: gold - orange - pink

Hawthorn *(Crataegus monogyna)*

Hawthorn, may, quickthorn or whitethorn is one of the commonest of British trees quickly establishing itself in both grassland and wood. Its slow growth and tangled spiny form makes it an ideal hedging plant for which it has been used down the centuries. Hawthorn flowers between late April and early June, though traditionally it signifies the quarter day of Beltane, the First of May, beginning of summer. The blossoms are creamy white, sometimes pink, and they lie densely along the top of the branches.

Hawthorn's primary importance is as a balance and regulator of the energies of the heart chakra, relieving stresses - whatever the quality or origin of that stress. It increases trust and the ability to give and receive love. It brings forgiveness, particularly of the self, and helps to cleanse the heart of negativity.

The heart chakra is the balance point and the centre of individual awareness. From this point the quality of the self is judged and how the self interacts and relates to all else in the world around it. The heart chakra is the standard by which the individual weighs and interprets all experience. As such, this energy centre needs to remain clear of stress and free from inappropriate beliefs if full potential is to be achieved in life.

As the central pivot of the energy structures of the body, the heart chakra affects every other channel and centre. Hawthorn, by balancing the heart chakra, can help to balance and align all the main energy centres.

Comment: Hawthorn, because of its blossom and time of flowering, is closely related to the fecund aspects of the Goddess energy. It also has close folklore associations with nature spirits and fairy beings. For such a small tree (although it can grow in woodland to over 50ft), hawthorn has a strong, powerful and characteristic presence and awareness.

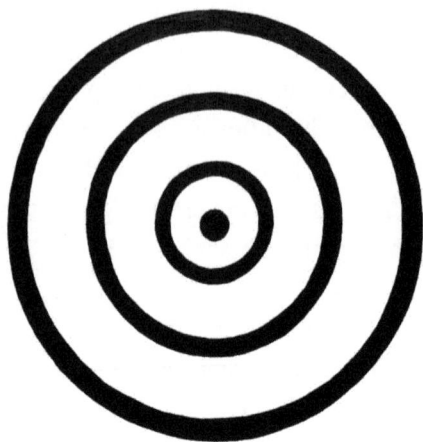

Hazel *(Corylus avellana)*

Keyword: skills

Colours: blue, gold

Chakras: 3, 5

Mantra: TOO-O'CHU. N'YAY-SHOO. JAY-SHAY (x3)

Note sequence: F# C

Colour sequence: gold - magenta - turquoise - indigo

Hazel *(Corylus avellana)*

Hazel is the earliest of British trees to come into flower. The long male catkins can be seen as early as January though it is usually February when they become heavy with yellow pollen. Hazel can grow to become a small tree of 30 ft, but it is more usually coppiced to harvest long, pliant rods or laid to make fast-growing hedging. It is usually short-lived but as a well-cared for coppice hazel has been recorded over a thousand years old.

The small, inconspicuous female flowers appear like small green barnacles with bright red stamens. Once ripened with wind-borne pollen they become a cluster of nuts, usually up to four together, each one enclosed in green leafy bracts.

Hazel is linked to the flowering of skills. It gives the ability to receive and communicate wisdom and so is excellent for both student and teacher. All forms of philosophy, teaching, information can be better assimilated and understood.

Because the mental body becomes better integrated with the physical body there is an ability to recognise those beliefs and ideas that hold the most usefulness and truth for the individual. The body's own intelligence and wisdom is involved here, which automatically brings more stability and focus into the present moment.

The throat chakra and a related centre where collar bones meet, is energised. This helps to clarify emotions and clear away unwanted debris, particularly those outdated beliefs about the self and problems with egotistical behaviour patterns. Hazel provides a communication doorways to many different levels of energy, particularly those relating to the spirits of earth and plants.

It is worth working with hazel when there is any uncertainty about direction of work or when ideas fail to give the necessary answers. All forms of mind-work from study to bardic inspiration to memorising, can be helped with this spirit energy.

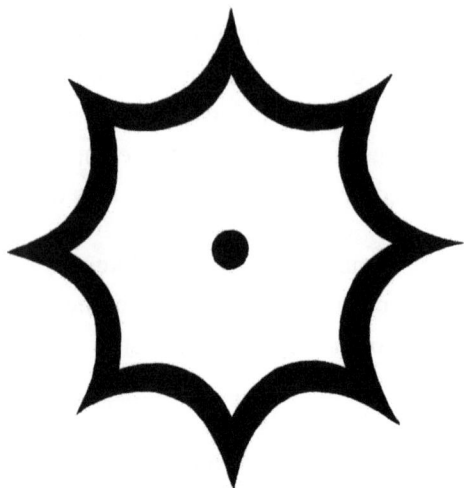

Holly *(Ilex aquifolium)*

Keywords: power of peace

Colour: pink

Chakra: 4

Mantra: T'SHAY TOE CHOOL

Note sequence: A C C D

Colour sequence: red - white - green - blue

Holly *(Ilex aquifolium)*

Few people are unable to identify the holly tree with its dark green glossy, evergreen leaves edged with sharp spikes. Holly will grow anywhere except excessively damp soil, and its well-protected leaves can withstand harsh conditions. Holly is common in hedgerows, often having been used in the past both as an effective barrier to animals and as a year-round guide in accurate siting of straight plough furrows. Male and female flowers grow on separate trees. Both bear small, waxy, white, four-petalled, sweet-scented flowers in May or early June. The fertilised female flowers swell to become the familiar red berries, loved by birds throughout the winter months. Holly grows in woodland as an under-storey tree able to tolerate low levels of light. It is very slow-growing and has a very fine, dense, white wood.

Holly is a spiritual guide and a balance for the mind. It helps clear away disturbances from the past that may cloud judgement. It encourages discrimination, balance and justice to develop.

The essence can help one to deal with panic, that loss of control linked to a sense of insecurity. Loneliness, the need for others, or dissatisfaction with oneself, the need for security, is addressed as is unhappiness, which again depends upon the sense of security, comfort and contentment. The Liver, Triple Warmer and Bladder meridians are all helped at this level.

The brow chakra is calmed. Irritability and noise at mental levels are reduced. Deep peace is given a chance to surface and communication processes are improved. This reduces friction in the system, calming everything right down. There is better appreciation of the quality of life-energy within the body, and this allows a more accurate picture of safety and risk in one's surroundings, increasing the ability to be flexible and cope with situations, turning them to advantage.

The higher subtle bodies become better integrated which releases tension and allows deep healing and creativity to flourish. This new spiritual re-integration can effectively remove deep-seated spiritual trauma and shock.

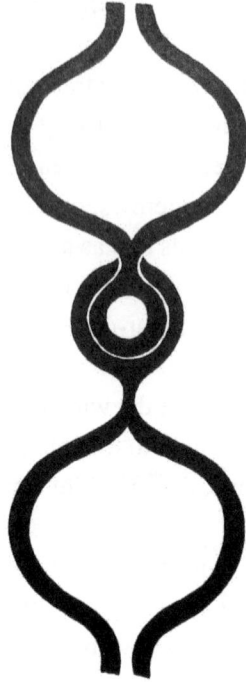

Holm Oak *(Quercus ilex)*

Keywords: negative emotions.

Colour: green

Chakra: 4

Mantra: KOO REE COW KOO

Note Sequence: C Eb *A *G *B Eb D

Colour Sequence: black - green - white - blue - red - black

Holm Oak *(Quercus ilex)*

The holly oak, or holm oak, is native to southern Europe. It has deep green evergreen leaves, slightly spiny when young, with paler undersides. It is a neat, dense looking tree often with multiple large boughs with the characteristic brown bark cracked into neat rectangles. It is a rather sombre-looking tree except where new growth appears a lighter yellow-green and a little later the long yellow catkins cover the tree in early summer. The acorns are rounder and more enclosed in their cups than the native oaks. Holm oak can grow to about 90ft (27m) and is often planted on exposed or seaward locations as it withstands salt winds and hot, dry conditions. It was introduced to Britain around 1500.

The essence focuses on the energy of personal space and personal expression. By activating personal creativity and a desire to assert oneself in a positive way in order to increase peace and harmony, holm oak helps to eliminate restlessness, impatience, frustration and all emotions that relate to thwarted expression. Thus negative feelings of anger, envy, greed and jealousy are dissolved. This directly strengthens the Bladder meridian allowing all such emotional disruptions and dissonances to be integrated and balanced into the system as a whole.

Holm oak helps to express personal power. There is a release of tension around the chest and back areas, and also in the lower abdomen as emotional and mental stresses are eased.

The sacral chakra is given greater energy and this helps to stabilise the life-energy in the body, also enhancing the sense of security and issues of worthiness and competence. This in turn allows the ego to become better aligned to the higher levels of consciousness within the individual.

Signature: The dark solidity of the tree emphasises its ability to calm and stabilise. The evergreen leaves suggest a continuity and stability of energy flow.

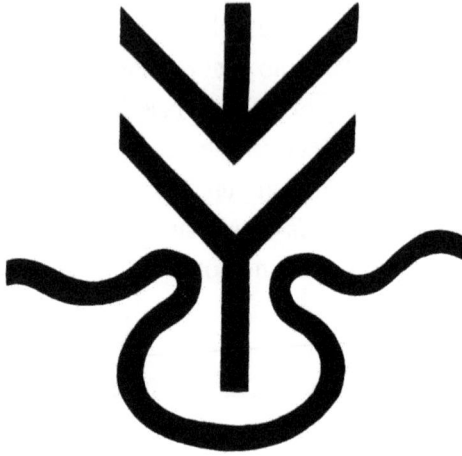

Hornbeam (*Carpinus betulus*)

Keywords: right action

Colour: orange, green

Chakras: 2, 4

Mantra: SHO CHEE BAA CHEE G'HUH'LUH SHO

Note Sequence: C B C# C# B B B C

Colour Sequence: like a dark night (non-defined darkness) - turquoise - blue -concentric rainbow colours

Hornbeam *(Carpinus betulus)*

Hornbeam is native to south-east England where hornbeam woodland still exists in places. Elsewhere it has been widely planted for timber and hedging. Hornbeam flowers in spring with both male catkins of green and female flowers at the end of branches emerging from young leaves with green bracts surrounding bright red styles. These ripen to form nutlets held within a three-lobed bract clustering at the end of branches. Hornbeam means 'hard wood' and it is one of the hardest and strongest of timbers formerly used for cogwheels, cutting blocks and wheel axles before iron became generally available.

Hornbeam essence creates the opportunity to clear those stresses that obscure our awareness of how we can achieve the greatest benefit from life. A flow of energy is deep, which can stimulate under-energised or stagnant areas and speed up internal communication systems. With these deep levels, available core belief systems and prime emotional stances can be transformed and directed towards a more dynamic, evolutionary and creative functioning. At the same time an increase of self-awareness and a sense of joy enables greater balance, harmony and growth. This can lead to clearer and more appropriate decision-making.

The Heart, Kidney and Triple Warmer meridians are affected and this helps to increase self-worth, creative security and the ability to serve within a collective framework. Anxiety and tension within the solar plexus chakra releases enabling a new creative balance of the mind and emotions, and this, too, increases the joy of life.

Hornbeam also clears away trauma from the deep energy systems of the body, particularly when these have been instigated through speaking out against consensus views. When personal expression has been repressed or censored hornbeam works at the throat chakra to increase confidence in speaking out and simultaneously grounds spiritual knowledge so that it can be of use. Hornbeam relates to cosmic power and energy as it manifests on the physical level.

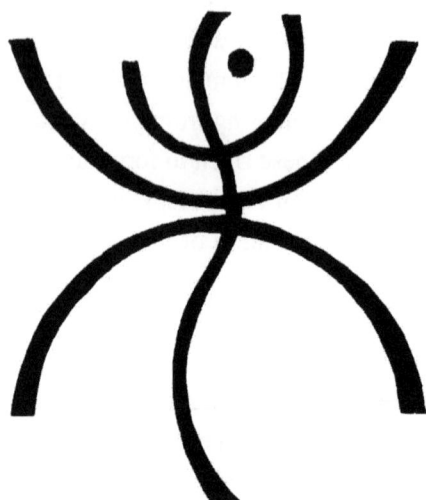

Horse Chestnut *(Aesculus hippocastanum)*

Keyword: agitation

Colour: blue

Chakras: 5, 6

Mantra: GAASH...T'HAASH DAA R. NAA Y

Note sequence: * Ab

Colour sequence: pink - red/orange - yellow

Horse Chestnut *(Aesculus hippocastanum)*

Horse chestnut could be found throughout central Europe before the last Ice Age but retreated to the high, moist valleys of the Balkan peninsula where it remained until the Turks took it to Istanbul in 1569. The tree was finally introduced into Britain in 1629. Horse chestnut is one of the largest flowering trees of the temperate world, its symmetrical, domed crown of hand-like leaves reaching to over 100 ft. (35m). The gnarled branches sweep upwards, then down then up again at the tips. The trunk is usually short and thick, always with a spiral to the right. Its wood is soft, easily worked but not strong enough for much significant timber uses, so it is primarily planted for its magnificent candles of white flowers in late spring.

The primary energy of the essence focuses on spiritual peace and the flow of intuition and information from one level to another. It provides the ability to utilise and accept transpersonal information, and from the Higher self for example.

There is an increased understanding and empathy with others which reduces the friction caused by great contrast. Feelings of intolerance and impatience can be lessened. Horse chestnut creates a flow between differing energies - rather than agitation. This releases emotional pressure from the Spleen and Bladder meridians. The root chakra, solar plexus chakra and crown chakra are affected. There is increased knowledge of what one requires and desires for physical well-being and balanced survival. There is a growth of wisdom that allows calm and clarity to develop and the ability to find one's personal space and life.

There is a regulation of energy flow between the crown and root chakras. This prevents any unnecessary build-up of energy and also grounds turbulence. This stress-free movement helps to bring about peace to agitated thoughts and repetitive patterns. The calm and balance improves mental functioning. Fears, anxieties and over-rational intellectual or obsessive thought are lessened bringing attention can dwell upon the deeper flows of intuition and the realisation that mind creates personal reality.

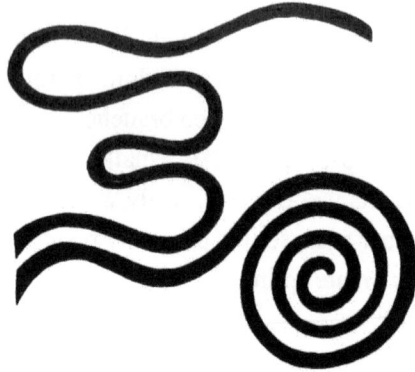

Italian Alder *(Alnus cordata)*

Keywords: protected peace

Colour: pink

Chakra: 4

Mantra: EYE JEE DHOO YO

Note Sequence: A B Eb* A

Colour Sequence: turquoise - orange - rainbow spectrum

Italian Alder *(Alnus cordata)*

The Italian alder, originating from Corsica and southern Italy, is the largest member of the family. In the wild it grows in dense thickets on damp ground, but it is tolerant of dry soil and is now much planted in towns and roadsides. It grows rapidly, has a tall, domed shape with bright, dense foliage up to 80 feet (24 metres). The leaves are heart-shaped, the catkins much fatter and larger than the native alder and the cones are heavier and more elongated.

This tree brings peace, love and protection for delicate energies. It can be helpful when there is either shyness or over-aggression. It provides courage and healing where new beginnings are needed.

Italian alder balances the Governor and Heart meridians to strengthen self-esteem and the feeling of being supported. Thus, it is for those who feel useless, unworthy, not valued, lacking in support, and so on. The soul body is also cleared of imbalances caused by guilt and this too, increases feelings of self-worth restoring energy to the physical being.

Peace and quiet enters the emotions restoring balance to the individual and the surroundings. It is able to heal emotional hurts and feelings of unworthiness and of being unloved.

At the finest levels of function Italian alder allows deep healing energies to enter from other dimensions. These are powerful protective levels of awareness that can neutralise polluting and aggressive vibrations.

Signature: The abundant upward growth and heart-shaped leaves.

Comment: Such an energy established in urban environments does much both at the physical and at subtle levels to cleanse the atmosphere. It is interesting to note that this tree has only begun to be planted in the last thirty years or so in Britain.

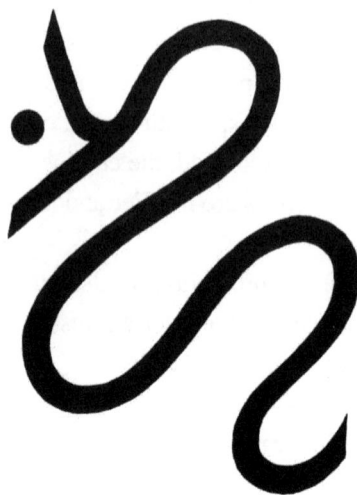

Ivy *(Hedera helix)*

Keyword: fear

Colour: green

Chakras: 3, 4

Mantra: KIJA. OH TRRR

Note sequence: E F Eb / E F Eb / E F Eb

Colour sequence: red, then: blue - gold - blue - gold - blue - gold...

Ivy *(Hedera helix)*

The ivy is one of the few plants that can thrive in deep shade. It can only very rarely be called a tree in its own right, though some old stems are as thick as tree trunks. Ivy is a climber, using walls and other plants for support as it reaches for height and sunlight. The triangular and five-pointed leaves are evergreen and often cover the floor of woods and copses. Ivy bears clusters of yellow flowers late in October, almost the last food for many insects. The black berries ripen over the next year.

As an essence ivy is very specific in its actions. Anxiety is the state it helps to resolve. Ivy specifically works with the chakra points at the wrists that help to ease hidden fears. Placing a few drops on these points will immediately reduce stress levels.

The heart chakra and its subtle channels, the nadis, are also strengthened bringing an increased calm and focus, as well as a greater sensitivity to one's surroundings. There is an increased ability to face fears and clearly examine those strong feelings for the underlying reasons. Ivy helps to rationally identify emotions and needs. By acting in this way stress is released and immune system function improves.

Ivy is an essential guide and protector both in working with tree spirits and confronting one's own inner fears successfully.

Signature: Lives in both dark and light. It flowers once it reaches the sunlight.

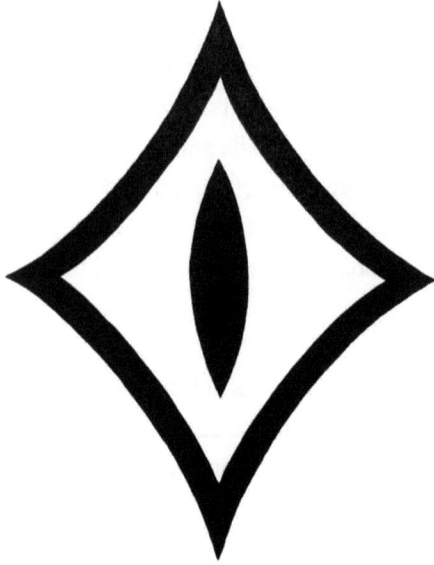

Judas Tree *(Cercis siliquastrum)*

Keyword: channelling

Colour: indigo

Chakra: 6

Mantra: GO PUH KAY DIE

Note Sequence: Eb D D C# C# C# E

Colour Sequence: Magenta - blue - orange

Judas Tree *(Cercis siliquastrum)*

Judas tree is native to dry, rocky places in western Asia and south-eastern Europe. The name probably derives from 'Judea Tree' in which area it is particularly frequent. Judas tree is a small, broad, spreading tree up to 33 ft. (10m). The leaves are kidney-shaped and before they fully emerge the flowers appear towards the end of May. The flowers are bright magenta-pink and grow singly and in bunches straight from the bark of twigs and trunk. It only really flourishes in the warmer parts of Britain, in sheltered spots.

As an essence, Judas Tree enables completely original thought, as if springing from nowhere. The seeds of new ideas arise from the deepest levels of the mind, where all available information has been stored and explored.

There is an openness and willingness to listen to one's own feelings. This can break patterns of repeating behaviour to do with past regrets enabling a new view of life. The Lung meridian is strengthened.

Communication and expression of personal opinion can be more direct, forceful and of a more practical nature. Nonetheless the essence also calms and soothes turbulent, passionate and angry states and enables rational, cool consideration of any situation involving the emotions. Throat chakra blocks are helped to clear in this way.

The development of channelling abilities is enhanced, together with the discrimination to discern the truthfulness within such thoughts.

Signature: The deep pink-magenta flowers (the colour of inspiration, universal energy and unity) spring straight from the bare bark.

Juniper *(Juniperus communis)*

Keyword: doorway

Colour: white

Chakras: 4, 5

Mantra: CHOO PIE MOW DHAA

Note Sequence: F# E Eb Eb D Eb *Eb

Colour Sequence: green - indigo - blue - turquoise - green

Juniper *(Juniperus communis)*

The juniper has the widest distribution of any tree, growing right across Europe, Siberia, Asia and America, from Atlantic to Pacific coasts. Juniper has a great many natural forms - it can resemble a gorse bush in shape, or can grow to become a neat conical tree up to about 20ft (6m). Male and female flowers grow on separate trees. In April and May they appear as small cone-like buds at the base of the needle-like leaves. Berries are dusty green and ripen to dark blue-purple in the second year. The berries are used to make gin and essential oils. Juniper has been used worldwide as an incense and a purifier of sacred space. It is said both to summon the ancestors and drive away harmful spirits.

Juniper brings a strength and revitalising energy to all levels of the body. It steadies the life-energy and allows it to move in those directions best suited to the individual. Sense of purpose and personal power to achieve goals is encouraged. It becomes easier to clarify intentions and make practical changes according to one's wishes.

Juniper essence helps to release us from the failures of the past. It relaxes the energy of the Circulation-Sex meridian, allowing us to accept and forgive mistakes and incorrect actions. Regret, remorse and jealousy are released. Those things that are really important and relevant are brought into focus. There is more confidence in one's own abilities and the capability to achieve one's own happiness. There is a relaxation, an acceptance of things as they are, and an increase in happiness and joy. Freedom from the weight of the past means the possibility of a completely new start to living.

There is a huge release of stress that has accumulated at the level of the sacral chakra. This is where stresses that cannot be immediately dealt with are buried. At very fine levels of the self there is increased discrimination, an innate intelligence that is able to see the hidden beginnings of things. In practice, this helps to reveal the distant past and how it has come to influence the present. Juniper offers us a way to link to the flow of our ancestor's history without being swayed by those events in any negative way.

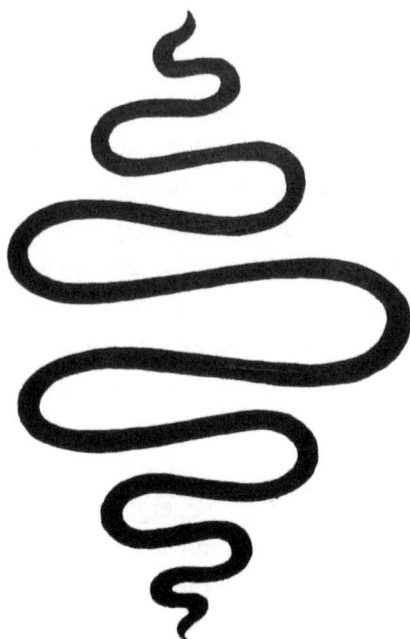

Laburnum *(Laburnum x watereri "Vossi")*
(Laburnum anagyroides)

Keywords: mental detoxification

Colour: orange

Chakra: 2

Mantra: G'HUT RRRI BHAA GAA SIGH

Note Sequence: C C C C# C C# C C# C# C C# C

Colour Sequence: orange - white - yellow - green - red

Laburnum *(Laburnum x watereri "Vossi")*
(Laburnum anagyroides)

Laburnum is native to the hill regions of central Europe. It is a small tree up to 30ft (9m) with smooth, olive green-brown bark and a tendency to arch over. In early summer yellow, pea-like flowers appear in long, pendulous strings. These ripen into green pods containing highly poisonous, shiny black seeds. The natural hybrid, Voss's Laburnum, arose in 1856 in the Tyrol and later (1865) also in Surrey, from *L. anagyroides* and *L. alpinum.* It is this variety that is most commonly planted for its spectacular flowers.

Laburnum creates the space and opportunity in which to allow the release of underlying imbalances, shock and traumas. By doing so it allows a growth of creative potential. There is a relaxation of muscular and nervous tension as the mental body is balanced and rigid belief systems or inappropriate concepts are abandoned. This allows a rapid detoxification of the system to take place. Likewise there is an increase in optimism, positivity and discrimination.

The throat chakra is stimulated and relaxation in this area will release tension, increase the ability to communicate and understand lessons, and listen to what is of use to the body systems - both physical and other forms of nutrition. The release of long-held stress memories brings a new balance and lightness to the emotions.

Signature: The fountain of yellow flowers and the somewhat weeping shape of the tree suggests letting go and the release of long held stresses. The dark seeds can be seen as the poisons released from the deep levels of the self. The heartwood is black and ebony-like whilst the sapwood is yellow – the darkness of the inner is changed to the joy of the outer.

Comment: Laburnum is an extremely graceful and beautiful little tree. However all parts and particularly the black seeds are extremely toxic causing sleepiness, convulsions, coma and death. Particular care needs to be taken when working with this spirit.

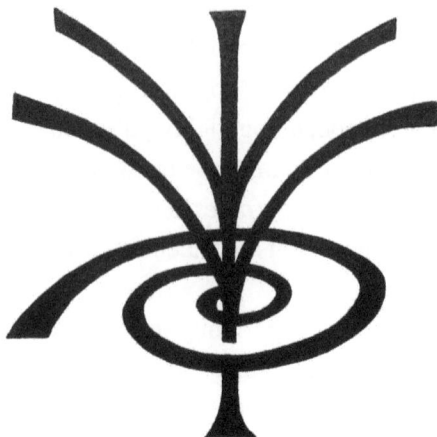

Larch *(Larix decidua)*

Keywords: will to express

Colours: orange, blue

Chakras 2, 5

Mantra: KEY BOO GO CHAI SO

Note Sequence: Eb F# Eb C Eb C#

Colour Sequence: white - blue/green - indigo - violet - white

Larch *(Larix decidua)*

Larch is the only deciduous conifer native to Europe. It is a mountain tree suited to long winters and short growing periods. Larch has a straight, single tapering trunk with long down-swung branches that make a narrow conical crown. It is fast growing yet can live for as long as 700 years. Female flowers are bright red and ripen into small cones that stay on the tree for many years. The male flowers are yellow and bud-like.

Larch helps to achieve balance through understanding the power of communication and the power of silence. It encourages wise judgement. In fact, larch introduces wisdom and awareness at every level so that it links to the creative, organising energies of the universe.

The main energies of this tree focus on the balance and expression of complementary energies particularly associated with the functions of the throat and sacral chakras, which can be characterised by the will to express the self and the desire to experience the outside of self.

The sacral chakra is affected, which controls and directs the physical energy towards expression and exploration of other beings in relationships. It motivates the joy for life and activate s healing creativity. Larch is an excellent essence for artistic activity bringing in both inspiration and the means to carry ideas into the world.

As a healer, larch can bring soothing and cooling energy to quite deep levels of hurt. There is greater acceptance of the physical levels of existence and the ability to let go and dissolve issues and experiences from the past.

Comment: Edward Bach used larch for those who felt they lacked the energy to succeed. Larch is an easily recognisable tree, often appearing untidy, unwell or even dying. But it knows what it is doing and is quite a friendly, very resinous, tree.

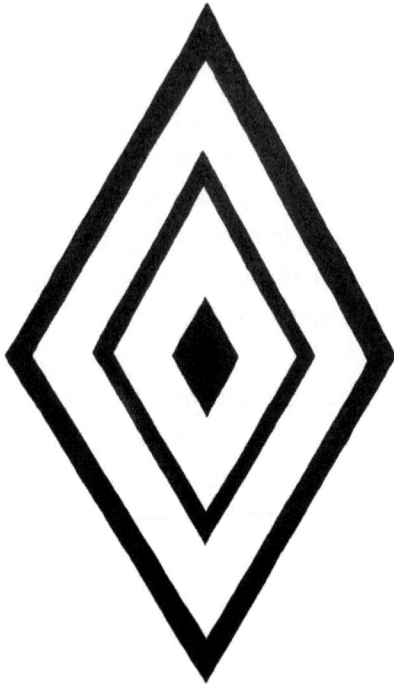

Lawson Cypress *(Chamaecyparus lawsoniana)*

Keyword: the path

Colour: green

Chakra: 4

Mantra: PAI VAU KHI

Note sequence: C* Bb G G
  (suffix *, denotes notes an octave above Middle C)

Colour sequence: violet - turquoise - yellow - black

Lawson Cypress *(Chamaecyparus lawsoniana)*

Lawson cypress has a very small natural range along 150 miles of north-west Pacific coastal America between North California and Oregon. It forms groups within the Redwood Forest. The buttressed trunk with thick reddish-brown fibrous bark reaches up to 200 feet or more. When in the open branches grow right from ground level. Lawson cypress was introduced into Britain in 1854 when seeds were sent to Lawsons nursery in Edinburgh. Some of the earliest trees are now over 100 feet. Although its form remains stable in the wild, once introduced into Europe it produced over 70 cultivars.

Lawson cypress activates those areas that are needed to identify correct action or the most appropriate direction in which to move. It brings energy into the base, sacral, solar plexus and brow chakras. In the root chakra it stimulates the required activity and discipline. The sacral chakra brings in the willingness to fulfil desires and to be flexible and creative in achieving them. The solar plexus is more closely linked to the energies of the higher self so that the individual's true needs can be communicated through intuition, dream and other symbolic forms. The essence also helps to clear out non-realistic, deluded or fantasised futures. The brow chakra maintains the overview and is enabled to clearly define in terms of thought, the 'feelings' activated in the lower chakras. All the subtle channels associated with these chakras are also cleared and activated.

In this way, Lawson cypress helps to bring the recognition of required actions; initiates change if that is appropriate; allows internal communication at the physical body-intelligence level; allows greater internal clarity to determine ones real needs, rather than those based wholly on intellect or fads.

This is a potent, powerful spirit. Learn to link with it and listen to it. Do not underestimate this tree just because of its domestic setting and ubiquity. Many trees have relied on humans to transport them around the world to take up residence in our closest surroundings. It may well be that they are of especial importance to our spiritual well being in urban communities.

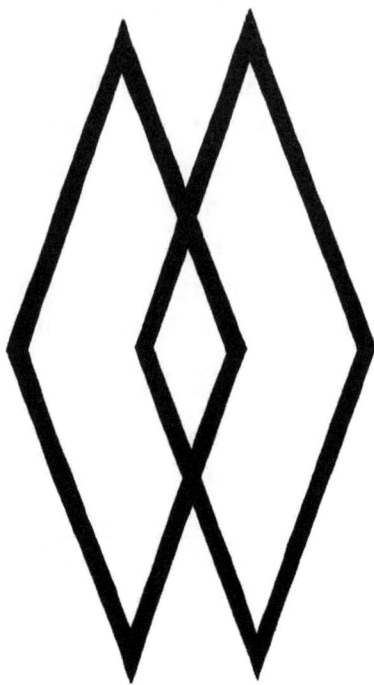

Leyland Cypress *(x Cupressocyparis leylandii)*

Keyword: freedom

Colour: green

Chakra: 4

Mantra: DEE RAY KEY TOO D'RR SHUH PIH

Note Sequence: F# C# F# F#

Colour Sequence: violet - blue - gold - white

Leyland Cypress *(x Cupressocyparis leylandii)*

This tree is a natural cross between the Nootka cypress fertilised by a Monterey cypress, which happened in Welshpool in 1888. In some respects, therefore, this is a truly native species, having its genesis in Wales! Leyland cypress quickly became popular as a hedging plant, combining the rapid growth of the Monterey and the hardiness of the Nootka. The trunk has numerous short branches from base to crown, both usually invisible through the thick, evergreen foliage. Small yellow male flowers appear in spring at the branch- tips. Female flowers are green and ripen later into small, green cones.

There is a sense of expansiveness and freedom. Where there has been anxiety and worry regarding the future, and where there is a lack of confidence and faith in positive outcomes, this essence re-energises the Spleen meridian to regain composure and trust.

It is possible to let go of unreal possibilities and delusions. A more stable and positive attitude is created with forgiveness, tolerance and compassion for oneself growing, together with an increased sense of humour. All this creates a sense of freedom and a space that feels comfortable. It helps to clear the head and shakes off muzziness. A useful essence for those who are frightened of being on their own or who are uncomfortable in their own company.

Signature: The structure of trunk and branches are kept hidden. The tree is planted as a fast-growing screen against noise, wind and to maintain privacy. Establishing personal boundaries. Both parent trees grow on the Pacific coast of America in spacious, wild surroundings.

Comment: It is interesting to note that this spontaneous generation of a new species occurred between two different, unrelated genera of tree at a time when the Victorian Age was fully occupied with the exploration of the 'green' energies of freedom, boundaries, discipline and power at the level of the individual, the society and the nation.

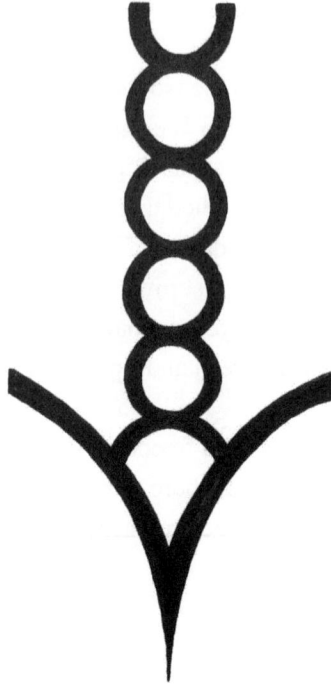

Lilac *(Syringa vulgaris)*

Keyword: spine

Colour: violet

Chakra: 7

Mantra: CO SHU KI……..CO SHU KI……..CO SHU KI

Sound Sequence: B C D F E D F

Colour Sequence: indigo - blue - green - orange - pink

Lilac *(Syringa vulgaris)*

Lilac was introduced to Britain in 1621 by John Tradescant, a prolific gardener of the time, from its native habitats of eastern Europe and Asia Minor. It now grows wild in many parts of the country. Lilac blossoms around May in large multi-flowered, strongly scented spikes of white, cream, lilac and purple. Lilac rarely grows tall, though it can reach 25ft (7.5m) and is usually a many-stemmed shrub with large, heart shaped leaves and a fibrous peeling bark.

The lilac essence mainly influences the spinal column. It works immediately on this area and so it is useful before any spinal adjustment, helping to stabilise any corrections, by increasing the energy flowing through the spinal channels and relaxing the supporting muscles. Lilac helps to correct posture and flexibility in the spine, largely through its influence on the subtle channels and major seven spinal chakras.

Because of the central role of the spine both physically and at subtle anatomical levels, lilac can be a useful adjunct to many corrective and evolutionary procedures. It will help restore balance throughout the system.

The lilac plant itself is thought to have a close link to many forms of nature spirits who use the energy of the lilac to elevate their own levels of awareness. This essence can also, then, be used to help us to attune more closely with these realms of awareness, both through the supportive energy link and also because lilac realigns so many fundamental energy systems within the body consciousness.

Signature: The heartwood of lilac is violet, reflecting the healing potential upon the spine and central energy channels. The sweet scented, small but substantial flowers cluster together and align into a tall spike, echoing the energy channels and centres of the body becoming integrated together.

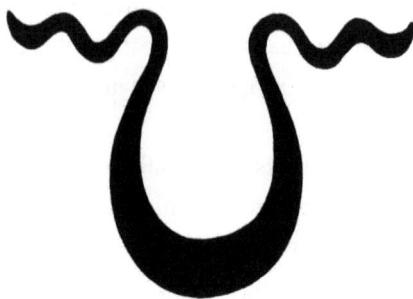

Lime *(Tilea x europa; Tilea platyphyllos; Tilea cordata)*

Keyword: development

Colours: yellow, green

Chakras: 3, 4

Mantra: DAA GI HAY. DAA GI HAY. DAA GI HAY.

Note sequence: C G E F Eb C. C GE F Eb C.

Colour sequence: orange - turquoise - indigo

Lime *(Tilea x europa; Tilea platyphyllos; Tilea cordata)*

The common lime is thought to be a cross between two other native species, the small-leaved and large-leaved limes. It is a tall tree that begins branching near the ground making a tall domed crown up to 130 ft (40m). The large-leaved lime can be distinguished by the fact it does not sprout from the base, unlike all other types.

Limes are long-lived trees, some of the oldest trees in Britain, and were one of the main woodland species. The soft wood is sweet scented and easily worked, the flowers are calming and relaxing, the inner bark is fibrous and can be woven into mats and rope.

Lime calms anxieties within the mind and helps to ease extremes of emotion, particularly when this is to do with making practical use of one's own developmental potential. Often the suppression of natural skills can seriously depletes our life-energy or directs the energy into negative, damaging behaviour patterns. The Gall Bladder meridian is helped to restore a positive balance to these strong emotions.

The solar plexus chakra and the eighth chakra, located above the head, are brought into action. This introduces the creative power necessary to move from one level of activity to another - whether that is a new awareness or a change of life-focus - in such a way that individual balance and the structure of the personality is maintained. Lime is thus useful in times of rapid growth or change. It can be of great benefit to those who are unable or unwilling to accept or use their higher faculties and subtle sensing skills. Doubts and fears of all sorts ease, and the familiar entrenched patterns of past behaviour are easier to overcome.

The lime is also known as the linden, its Germanic name. On the Continent the tree is still often found at the heart of the village as guardian and focus for the community. In the past lime would have been such a predominant woodland species and useful both medicinally and as a material resource.

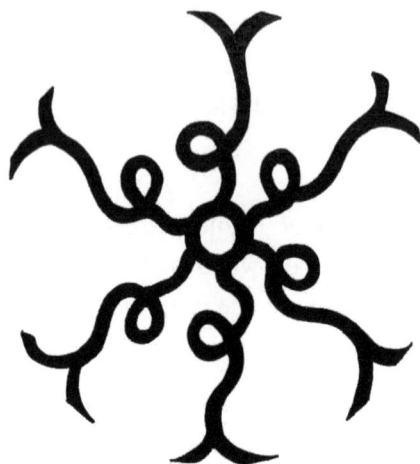

Liquidamber (Sweet Gum) *(Liquidamber styraciflua)*

Keywords: sweet tongue

Colours: orange, blue

Chakras: 2, 5

Mantra: TUH LUGOO TIT OW TU LUH

Sound Sequence: G *Eb *F# *Eb

Colour Sequence: blue - yellow - indigo - black - indigo

Liquidamber (Sweet Gum) *(Liquidamber styraciflua)*

This tree superficially resembles the Acer family, but its leaves are alternate rather than opposite. The leaves are strikingly large with five or seven distinct pointed lobes, the central, terminal lobe being a lot larger than the side lobes. Leaves are smooth and finely toothed turning to a range of magnificent colours in autumn, from oranges to reds to violets, purples and blacks. Liquidamber originates from Mexico and the southern United States and is famous for its aromatic gum resin that exudes from the trunk.

The energy of liquidamber is dynamic and passionate. It works primarily with the emotional drives that it is able to direct and mould in compassionate and creative ways. Liquidamber moulds raw emotional energy to bring the individual maximum emotional support and positive life-energy. Liquidamber strengthens the Governing meridian. It gives backbone - the courage of one's convictions. It helps to maintain personal energy integrity in situations where there is opposition to the individual expressing their own needs and opinions, preventing entrainment at any energy level, physical, electromagnetic or subtle.

The sacral chakra is a focus for this tree's energy. There is the desire to satisfy personal creativity, to manifest one's deepest wishes, to really get involved and dive into the fullness of living. Symptoms that express the blocking of the sacral chakra – emotional detachment, lack of feeling, boredom, rigidity, inability to relax – would all be eased with this tree essence.

Liquidamber also encourages a great ability to heal through communication. At the throat chakra (complementary energy centre to the sacral chakra), there is the possibility of using the voice with great skill - in such a way that a flow of loquaciousness, a 'sweet tongue', can heal the body, calm the mind and nourish the spirit. It also helps to balance the relationship of the individual to the object of love by relaxing the natural fear of opening too much, of giving too much away, of risking failure, so that a more spontaneous behaviour is possible.

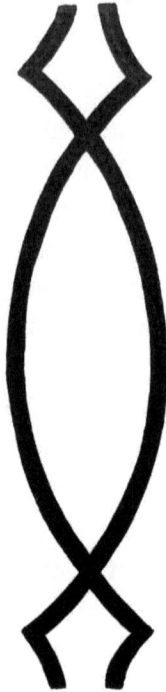

Lombardy Poplar *(Populus nigra 'italica')*

Keyword: aspiration

Colour: indigo

Chakras: 3, 6

Mantra: BEE PIE GHOO JOE FUH VOO

Note Sequence: Ab C# E C Ab E

Colour Sequence: white - yellow - black - indigo - orange

Lombardy Poplar *(Populus nigra 'italica')*

Lombardy poplar is a natural form of the southern European black poplar found in Northern Italy and first introduced into Britain in the middle of the 18th century by Lord Rochford who planted it at St. Osyth Priory, Essex. It is the male trees, bearing large red catkins in April, that tend to be planted in Britain. Lombardy poplar can reach 130ft (40m) with a sweeping, elongated oval profile. In the USA, where it is commonly planted, the hot autumns turn the trees into stunningly beautiful, golden towers.

The main quality of this essence is the understanding of intuitive processes. It helps to discriminate between information from different sources, sharpening the intellect so that it can make sense of intuitive feelings. The sacral chakra is particularly energised so as to allow an expression of personal creativity that can release and reveal one's personal goals and ambitions. The creative flow when released will then naturally follow a very individual and empowering path.

The subtle bodies, particularly the Causal and Spiritual bodies (both very fine, non-personality based aspects of the self), are also motivated along the same lines. The Causal body is enabled to access karmic influences that directly influence the current life. There are certain patterns of behaviour that we carry with us and, unless we consciously let go of them, they tend to become entrenched, even though they are outmoded or prove continually to be unsuccessful strategies. With the Spiritual body it brings us a better understanding of the illusory strength of emotional reactions. Not that emotions are not real - simply that they occur much like the weather in the world occurs.

Lombardy poplar essence can help to reveal the most profound levels of communication from deep time (the edges of space and time as we perceive them), through the unique expression of the personality. The essence can reveal what is motivating our personal choices, our patterns of behaviour, and what activity naturally supports the flow of our unique life-energy.

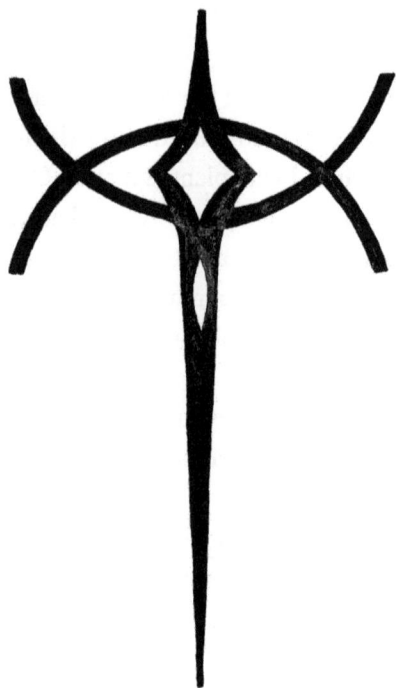

Lucombe Oak *(Quercus hispanica "Lucombeana")*

Keywords: creative energy

Colours: orange, violet

Chakras: 2, 7

Mantra: PODE H'RRRRUH K'RRRRUH K'RRRRUH

Note Sequence: C *F# *G C C# Eb Eb *G

Colour Sequence: yellow - orange - yellow - white - turquoise - red with green flashes

Lucombe Oak *(Quercus hispanica "Lucombeana")*

Lucombe oak is named after an Exeter nurseryman who found a natural cross between turkey oak and cork oak. When the two original hybrids produced acorns in 1792 they were grown and distributed. There are many forms, but the common Lucombe oak is fully evergreen with shiny dark green leaves and pointed teeth and has a slightly corky bark with keel-like swellings on the trunk near the branches. Other types are closer to one parent or the other with lighter, thick corky bark or not fully evergreen. It can be found in parks and gardens throughout Britain but is most common in Devon, especially in Exeter itself. Like other oak it produces clusters of yellow, male catkins in spring and female flowers that ripen into acorns enclosed in a mossy green cup during the second year.

The focus of this tree is a life-supporting creativity bringing inspiration and ideas. The crown chakra is able to infuse the mind with the awareness of evolutionary activity. The mental body is thus energised and is enabled to act with a greater commitment for change and growth. Any state of lethargy, lack of commitment or confusion can be helped with Lucombe oak.

There is increased tolerance and kindness born of wisdom and compassion. Stressful and life-harming beliefs are able to be released by an infusion of non-aggressive awareness. This can be deeply healing.

Individual consciousness, encapsulated within the fourth, or astral, body is helped to remove fears relating to personality, past lives and life-purpose. There is a clarity of mind with a greater ability to focus and learn from experience.

At its subtlest Lucombe oak reveals the finest levels of inspiration, where creativity and creative intelligence spring from the unmanifest, absolute nature of reality. With this quality of energy accessible the full potential can be brought forward in a dynamic and energetic manner before it becomes diluted and constrained by limitations. Lucombe oak embodies creativity, creative intelligence and manifestation of the creative urge.

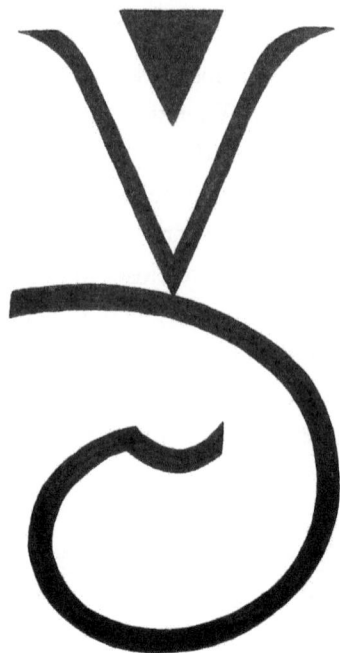

Magnolia *(Magnolia x soulangeana)*

Keyword: restlessness

Colour: green

Chakra: 4

Mantra: RU KOO AA RU

Note sequence: F G Eb Bb F

Colour sequence: gold - turquoise - white - dark blue

Magnolia *(Magnolia x soulangeana)*

An open-branched, short-trunked tree growing to 25 ft, magnolia is well-loved for its flowers during April and May. As buds, they resemble steady white candle flames and as flowers they bear a similarity to lotuses or pink and white doves alighting on the branches.

Magnolia is a large family with members native to North America and China where different species have been used medicinally from protection against malaria to lowering of blood pressure. This common variety is a cross between two Chinese species grown near Paris in the 19th century.

Magnolia helps with the understanding of the healing process, releasing fears to increase calm and the inherent healing potential within the self.

Stomach and Governor meridians become activated to remove feelings of vulnerability and lack of clarity. Helps where there is an unsettling restlessness in which nothing satisfies.

The heart chakra and its nadis are cleansed of stress and trauma allowing a greater freedom of emotional expression and relaxation. The crown chakra is enabled to clarify true identity and the validity of past and present experiences.

When there are major life-decisions to be made and a need to clarify direction and what should be done, the causal subtle body, the fine level of awareness that patterns how we are, is energised. This helps when there are difficult choices. Heart and mind are brought into equilibrium and this allows calm and happiness in which to make the correct decisions.

Signature: The open, relaxed growth; the flowers resemble the subtle colours of the lotus, and so therefore the chakras.

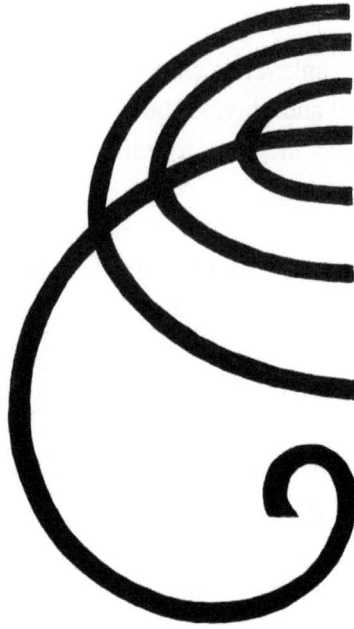

Manna Ash *(Fraxinus ornus)*

Keywords: happy with oneself

Colour: pink

Chakra: 4

Mantra: JAY GURRA JEE TOO BURRA GUH' GURRA

Note Sequence: G C C C G E F E D C

Colour Sequence: green - fading to darkness

Manna Ash *(Fraxinus ornus)*

The manna ash was introduced into Britain in 1700, though it is usually grown as a graft on the common ash. It is native in Asia and southern Europe. It is a small, round-crowned tree to 80 ft (24m). The leaves are densely packed and of similar form to common ash though shorter and less pointed. It is the flowers of manna ash that are its most noticeable feature, starting off as bright green clustered buds that open in May or June as creamy-white scented flowers that elongate into masses of feathery threads.

Manna ash works primarily with healing the emotions. It helps to bring the recognition of what is needed to establish peace. It also allows an openness and honesty regarding one's true nature and what are the main motivating desires. This in itself can release deep blocks to self-expression.

Seeing more clearly one's true nature and being honest with oneself increases the energy available throughout the entire meridian system. The Governing meridian is strengthened. The Heart meridian is also given energy to clear emotional blocks from the heart. Manna ash increases self-worth and allows a process of self-acceptance to bring purification and transformation.

Manna ash helps to sort out unresolved issues. It will also help to integrate the subtle bodies and this reduces aggravation and destructive tendencies caused by conflicts of emotion. Relationships of all kinds are seen in a wider and more constructive perspective.

The healing of subtle body imbalances and disturbances leads to an easing of mental stress. A quiet, creative level of consciousness is more easily accessed from which to draw greater healing.

At its finest levels manna ash allows a flow of wisdom and healing creativity from the level of pure consciousness, the source of all.

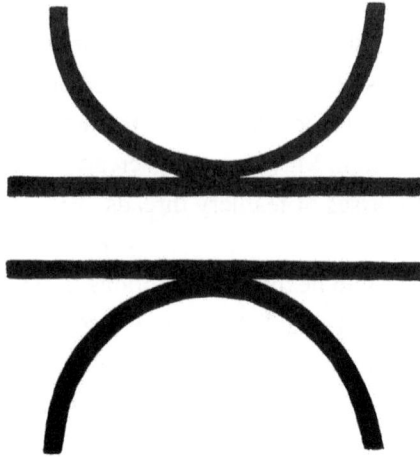

Medlar *(Mespilus germanicus)*

Keyword: boundless

Colours: red, gold

Chakra: 3

Mantra: BUY NYEE SHA HUW NYEE

Note Sequence: F# C E C *F

Colour Sequence: blue - pink - white - dark turquoise - yellow - indigo

Medlar *(Mespilus germanicus)*

A small, gnarled tree to 20ft originally from the Caucasus. Its fruit was popular with Greeks and Romans, the latter who introduced the medlar into Britain. The leaves are large and downy with a single white wild rose-like flower at the end of each twig in summer. The scent is strong and not entirely pleasant.

Medlar fruit is unusual - it doesn't fall from the tree and is only edible when it is over-ripe - very often after a few frosts or having been picked for a few weeks. Both flower and fruit are unmistakable.

Medlar essence energises personal core patterns, one's *raison d'etre*, and helps them to develop into physical and practical expression. Increased motivation, enthusiasm and drive. There is a feeling of boundless energy to achieve goals.

The sacral chakra and solar plexus chakra are strengthened. There is an increase in joy and happiness, and a deep 'gut feeling' of safety and security. Creativity and the finest levels of self-awareness are more easily grounded into the practical desire to manifest and make real. Personal needs and neuroses are put into a broader context of the underlying enfoldment of the universal energies. Small selfishness is tempered by a feeling of secure expansiveness.

There is an expansion of strength, humour, brightness and creative intelligence that affects both the emotions and the spirituality.

Signature: The fruits remain attached to the tree: security, confidence. Adverse conditions only serve to 'blet' or ripen, the internal sweetness.

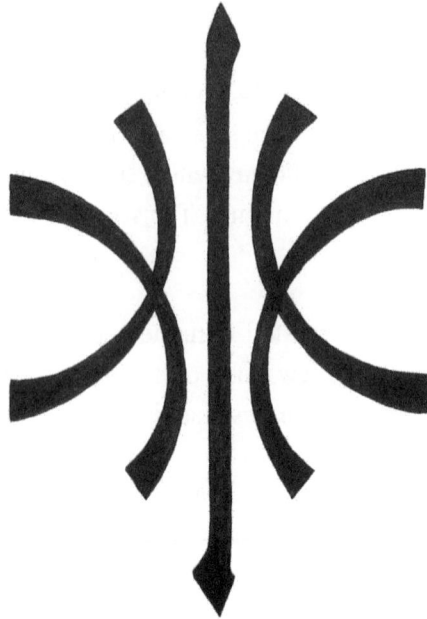

Midland Hawthorn *(Crataegus laevigata)*

Keyword: expansion

Colours: red, green

Chakra: 4

Mantra: D'HAA

Note Sequence: Ab G Eb F# G Ab

Colour Sequence: white - violet - blue - orange - yellow - black

Midland Hawthorn *(Crataegus laevigata)*

A less common variety of hawthorn in the wild, though more widely planted in gardens for its blossom, the midland hawthorn grows on heavier soils. It can be identified by a more fluted, twisted trunk and has leaves that are more rounded and less indented then common hawthorn. Although its flowers can be white, the varieties chosen for planting are pink or deep red. "Paul's Scarlet" is the richest of reds with double petalled flowers.

The essence brings the quality of spaciousness and deep peace to relationship issues. The small selfish viewpoint is broadened out and relaxed to allow a calm overview.

Much energy focuses around the heart and its subtle centres, especially those to do with directing the heart energy into spiritual growth. The temptation to over-emotionalise and "go overboard" on spiritual quests is balanced so that spiritual aspects can become integrated into everyday life.

There is an increased desire to live life to the full, to enjoy, learn, use and discover as much of life as is humanly possible. This extra energy is an antidote for the weak-willed or those who fear exploration, and yet helps to moderate reckless or impulsive tendencies. With this enthusiasm to grow and investigate for oneself there comes an awareness of innovative concepts and inspirations which allow for personal expansion.

Signature: The rich red blossom energises the senses at a time of year when all life is expanding and growing into summer.

Comment: Like many other species, the hawthorns seem to focus their group energy on a similar area of life. Here it is primarily the heart and aspects of relationship, growth, personal freedom and expansion that can be seen in hawthorn, Glastonbury thorn and midland hawthorn.

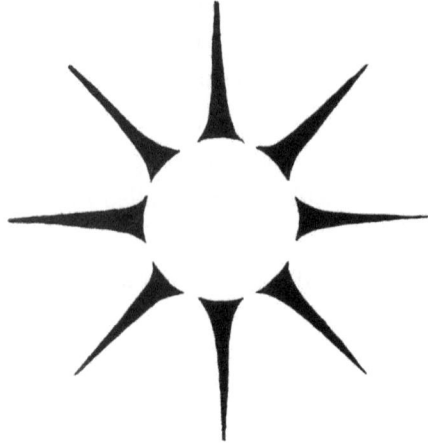

Mimosa *(Acacia dealbata)*

Keyword: sensitivity

Colours: yellow, blue

Chakras: 3, 6

Mantra: RNAA SHAY BOO, RNAA SHAY BOO.

Note Sequence: D *G G A

Colour Sequence: green - blue - blue with white veining - yellow

Mimosa *(Acacia dealbata)*

Also known as the silver wattle, this tree originally comes from S.E. Australia and Tasmania where it grows in mountain gullies and on the banks of streams. It is quite widely planted in southern Europe but cannot survive cold winters or exposed conditions. The mild climate in the South West of England means that it is quite a common sight to see the small, bright yellow, fragrant clusters of flowers in January and February, just after the evergreen blue-green feathery leaves begin a new growth. Mimosa can grow to 65ft. The yellow pompom like flowers are often used in flower arranging.

Mimosa increases the sensitivity of the nervous system to internal body stimuli. This helps to improve the flow of energy and information between different systems, encouraging a smoother functioning.

The essence affects the Small Intestine meridian and the Large Intestine meridians, particularly with those issues to do with the assimilation of energies at a physical level, as well as ideas and information at a mental level and the ability, at whatever level, to let go and release what is not required. This can be of benefit in any cleansing or detoxifying process.

There is a beneficial effect on the emotions, with an increased sense of peace.

A minor chakra in the upper throat is stimulated and this gives the will to express one's thoughts and to speak up.

The mental body is better balanced so that greater information and clarification can be received from the intuition. The subtle, causal body is steered more towards self-motivation and the power to express one's universal nature in an individual way.

Signature: The delicate leaves and globe-like clusters of flowers. Yellow: clarity, mental organisation, identification processes.

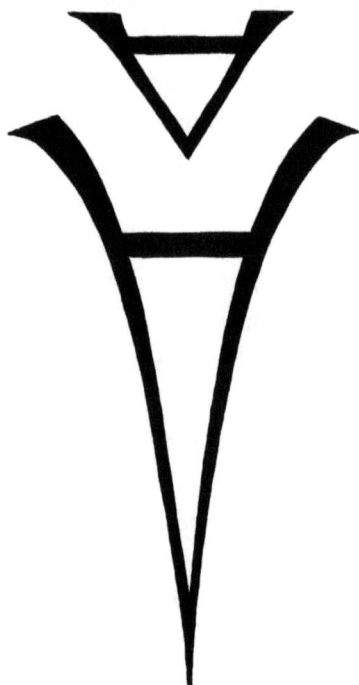

Monkey Puzzle Tree *(Araucacia araucana)*

Keywords: fierce compassion

Colours: red, pink

Chakras: 1, 4

Mantra: SHOW KLE KAA

Note sequence: G Eb G G F# D B

Colour sequence: orange - yellow - pink - magenta - orange

Monkey Puzzle Tree *(Araucacia araucana)*

The Chile pine, known throughout Britain by its Victorian name the 'monkey puzzle tree', is native to a small area around the Andean mountain, Volcan Llaima. Its name derives from the Araucanian peoples who depend quite heavily on the large seeds as a food source. Five seedlings were brought back to Kew Gardens in 1795 by botanist Alexander Menzies who had never seen a specimen in the wild. In 1884 more seeds were brought from Chile and the major plantings took place then. The tree is unmistakable with each branch completely covered in overlapping, dark green, rigid leaves. The monkey puzzle can grow to 80ft (24m) and has a neat, domed crown often losing its lower branches but is fairly short-lived, averaging 100 years.

The monkey puzzle tree is characterised by action that is expressed through caring, understanding and compassion. It will calm aggression but still allows that energy to be manifested in a creative, forceful way. The essence is strongly energising, earthing and protecting from negativity.

One particular characteristic of this tree is that it enables a great understanding and the experience of joyfulness in witnessing the continuous cycles of change upon the planet – sunrise to sunset, day and night, heat and cold, summer and winter, activity and stillness. The perception of the underlying stability and continuity of awareness running throughout, expands the sense of time and space. This enlarged view helps the release of tension and anxiety. Talking to the long memory of the planet, and becoming enfolded within the story.

The way each leaf overlaps from the last suggests the overlapping and continuous cycles of growth and time. The nuts were the main sustaining food crop of the Araucanian people: a fierce tree providing plentiful harvests.

In Britain, the monkey-puzzle is synonymous with Victorian park and garden planning, and with that period's rather fusty provincialism. It takes a fresh vision to go beyond this accreted, received view to see the tree in the context of its own energy.

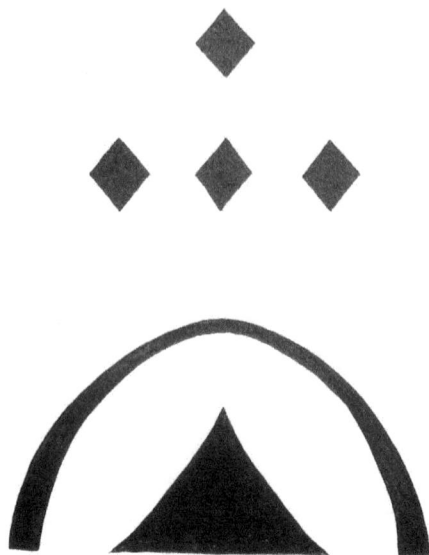

Monterey Pine *(Pinus radiata)*

Keyword: connectedness

Colour: red, violet

Chakra: 7

Mantra: YEAR(uh) EH TURR(uh) HO SHAY

Note sequence: Bb F .. Bb. F .. (repeated)

Colour sequence: blue - yellow - blue

Monterey Pine *(Pinus radiata)*

During the Ice Age, pines grew in the southern parts of North America. When the ice melted, a few small pockets remained only on the Monterey peninsula in California where it is a low-growing, wind-blown tree. Monterey pine was introduced to Britain in 1833. Here it grows rapidly. With dense triple needles of grass green and the ability to thrive in salt and windy exposed locations at low altitudes, it quickly became established as a windbreak.

In Britain the tree can grow twice as fast as normal, sometimes throughout the whole year, and has reached a height of over 180 ft. In spring male flowers are found in long spikes at the base of new shoots, heavy with yellow pollen. Female flowers are red-brown and found at the tops of new shoots. The ripened cones can remain on the tree for up to 30 years.

Monterey pine helps the removal of deep stresses from the system - particularly those relating to speaking out against perceived injustices and the failure to speak out when necessary. It becomes easier to be happy in one's own company and self-sufficient. There is an increasing sense of purpose and ease with the self and the surroundings. A calm and clarity reaches the emotions.

There is a sense of physical well-being - getting in touch with the body. There is an increased confidence in the physical body. Subtle perceptive abilities are enhanced with the possibility of past-life information and an increased understanding of ideas, concepts and other energy planes.

The release of deep-seated stresses help to promote self-expression and artistic creativity, so this essence can be useful when there are artistic blocks. The new flow of energy brings a sense of deep peace and connectedness to everything. There is a balance between active and passive modes of behaviour, between aggression and submission and between male and female polarities. This extra confidence relaxes preconceptions and rigidity of beliefs.

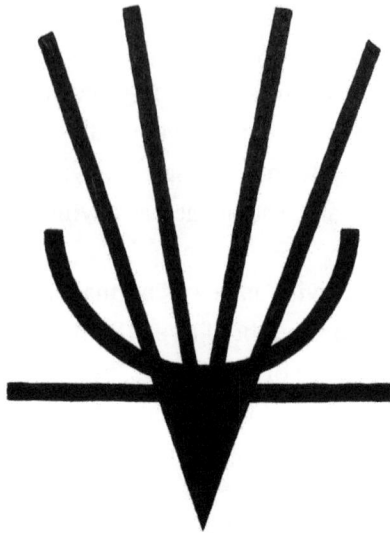

Mulberry (Black Mulberry) *(Morus nigra)*

Keyword: wrath

Colours: dark-red, magenta

Chakra: 1

Mantra: TEE SHOOED NYAI NYAA

Note sequence: B A B G

Colour sequence: indigo - violet

Mulberry (Black Mulberry) *(Morus nigra)*

A small, gnarled, rough looking tree with large heart-shaped leaves. In May it produces green male and female catkins, the latter which ripen into large, rich red fruit. Perhaps originating from the Middle East, mulberry was brought west by the Greeks and Romans. It has been grown in Britain since 1550. The Chinese variety is white mulberry upon which silkworms feed. Both species have medicinal properties.

Here there is emotional healing. Mulberry brings compassion, peace and a necessary detachment from the source of pain. It works through the Spleen meridian, Liver meridian and Circulation-sex (Pericardium) meridian. It can be for those who decry any views that differ from their own and who will not see deeper truths, and for those who are jaded and cynical about the world – dominant, worldly-wise cynics.

For those attached to a painful situation or event and carry within them great remorse, Mulberry helps to heal the energy link and brings peace. There is freedom from past pain and remorse.

It changes the energy of anger towards more constructive ends where it can be mastered and fully expressed through understanding the truth of the underlying situation. It will allow full expression of feelings but helps to curb excessive wrathfulness.

The solar plexus chakra is activated to protect fine levels of emerging awareness and to manifest these in practical ways. The mind is given a degree of energy that enables inspirational concepts and ideas to find creative expression - particularly when the ideas seem to be coming from beyond personal experience.

On a universal level this essence acts as a pathway to some of the super-physical consciousnesses of the solar system, the loving intelligence that directs and oversees the creative processes in each area of the physical cosmos.

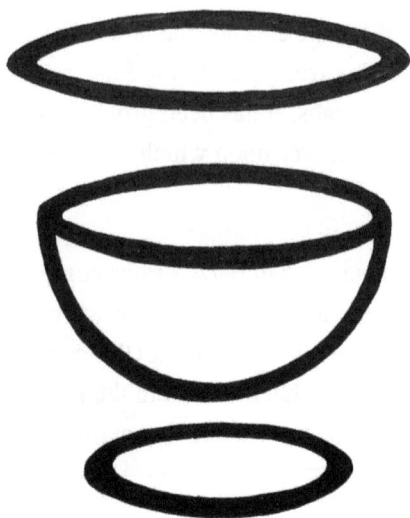

Norway Maple *(Acer platanoides)*

Keywords: healing love

Colours: gold, pink

Chakras: 2, 3

Mantra: SHIK EYE RIP AY RIH

Note Sequence: F Ab Ab F# F# G G F

Colour Sequence: green field with slow pulsing pink points - yellow - white

Norway Maple *(Acer platanoides)*

Norway maple is a native in Europe apart from Britain and the Lowlands. It is a large deciduous tree with a short bole and a wide-domed crown reaching to 90ft. Bright green leaves are typically maple-shaped and turn bright yellow in autumn. In spring, before the leaves, it produces a profusion of surprisingly bright yellow-green flowers in erect bunches. Introduced into Britain in 1683, Norway maple is now very common and easily self-seeds in sandy soil. It is also popular as a town tree, partly because of its rapid growth when young.

Primarily healing on emotional levels, this essence brings love, acceptance, healing and nurturing energy to states of emotional shock and trauma.

The Triple-Warmer meridian and Liver meridian are cleansed to restore a sense of lightness and happiness.

The crown chakra is able to access healing and creative energy, and this flows down into the body to enable one to take back control of situations where there is a feeling of powerlessness. There is clarity in accepting the reality of circumstances and working to find ways of working within them.

The emotional and spiritual bodies are aligned and this will help the most subtle aspirations of the personality guide the feeling level towards appropriate activity and direction.

There is an increased understanding of situations and this encourages relaxation and particularly release of tension at the solar plexus. Fears and anxiety ease, joy and comfort increase.

As this process of relaxation and empowerment continues it is more possible to access deeper levels of personal potential where it is brought to awareness through inspiration and imagination. There is an ability to harmonise with universal qualities of compassion and healing, aligning to a creative flow of energy that creates freedom and healing.

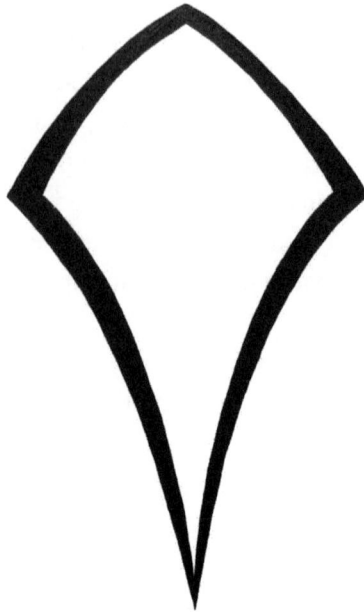

Norway Spruce *(Picea abies)*

Keyword: trust

Colours: orange, blue

Chakras: 2, 5

Mantra : D'HIH HURAT. BOW BAA

Note Sequence: B A G* G* G*

Colour Sequence: yellow - gold - white - green

Norway Spruce *(Picea abies)*

Norway spruce is a mountain tree of highland Europe, growing from the Balkans to Scandinavia. Before the last Ice Age the tree grew in Britain but disappeared until it was reintroduced in the early years of the 16th century. The young trees are familiar to us as the Christmas tree, but left to mature it can become a large timber tree up to 130ft (40m) living for about two hundred years.

Change is the one fundamental quality of life. It is the one constant in the universe of energy. Understanding this allows change to happen, and along with it comes transformation and purification. Letting go and knowing that you will fall into something more interesting is the essence of Norway spruce. The acceptance that everything that happens is the potential for new beginnings helps us to focus on what we have rather than what we may lose.

The Triple Warmer meridian is particularly stimulated. This allows a flow of protecting energy to circulate throughout the whole being. The reduction of fear and tension eases internal communication and so reduces stress.

With this tree energy comes delight in exploring new avenues, a sense of ease, a natural happiness and an ability to share at the level of the feelings and the senses. This change is focused on the activity of the sacral chakra. When unbalanced or over-energised, this energy centre can create a hedonism or profound selfishness, but with Norway spruce it is possible to remain true to one's own feelings without insisting that your point of view is the only right way to live. There is confidence to acknowledge personal experience without denigrating other's feelings.

The Etheric body, so important to the integrity of the body as a whole, is helped to remove the problems caused by aggressive emotional patterns. Fragmented parts of the self are unified in self-healing. The mind becomes clearer and it is easier to communicate information. At the finest spiritual level comes the ability to access deep intuitive flows of inspirational knowing, and possibly even the communication of profound teachings.

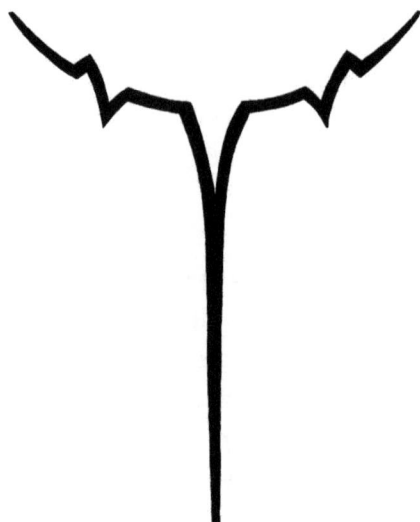

Oak *(Quercus robur, Quercus petraea)*

Keyword: manifestation

Colour: red

Chakra: 1

Mantra: DOW TAA BEY PEY DHEY

Note sequence: Bb Bb C Bb E

Colour sequence: red - yellow - blue - white - indigo - black

Oak *(Quercus robur, Quercus petraea)*

The two native oaks in Britain can be identified by form and habitat where they haven't cross-bred many times. The common oak, also called the English oak or pedunculate oak, favours lower land and heavier soils. The sessile oak prefers wetter climates and lighter soils. The common oak has leaves with no stalks but acorns with stalks, whilst the sessile oak has leaves with long stalks and acorns with none. The oak flowers as it opens its leaves. The male catkins are yellow green and cluster together soon becoming long like knotted strings. The female flowers are small buds at the branch ends, green with bright red anthers. The English oak can reach 115 ft (35m) and the sessile oak grows to 130 ft (40m).

The energy of the oaks in general has to do with the ability to manifest, to bring forth, maintain and balance reality. Steady growth and drawing out potential from where it is hidden from sight can be accomplished with oak. The Heart meridian is brought into balance, which relaxes and expands the emotions.

Many of the subtle energy centres and channels of the body are given a boost of energy and the eleventh chakra above the head is activated. This helps to integrate the personality located in time-space with the transpersonal collective, Higher self or soul group, making it easier to understand and direct the purpose of lifetime activities.

The Earth star chakra is strongly activated. Security, belonging, taking one's place, stability, practicality, all rely on a firm grounding link that this chakra supplies. Keeping a body well and functioning requires the will to exist on this planet, here and now. Oak provides this motivation. The spiritual state brought about by oak spirit is profoundly internalised, involuted and dwells at the unmanifest levels of creation. Oak essence aids in the absorption and integration of these very deep, hidden energy levels from the primal sources of being. The oak spirit funnels it through the desire for growth and expansion into physical dimensions of reality, and will encourage delight in expressing the energy of growth in as many ways as possible.

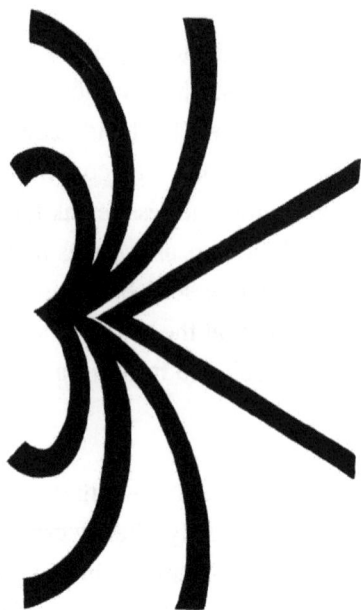

Olive *(Olea europea)*

Keyword: valour

Colours: red, gold

Chakras: 1, 3

Mantra: MRRUH TOO J'HEY TOO

Note Sequence: A Bb Eb D D Eb C

Colour Sequence: gold - blue - white - red

Olive *(Olea europea)*

The olive is the most important crop tree of the Mediterranean area. It is a cultivar that derives from its wild relative, *Olea sylvestris*, a smaller bushier tree with spiny stems and smaller leaves and fruits.

Olive's energy benefits those who have great passions and strong drives. It gives the ability to be able to direct these strong desires in a creative and life-enhancing direction enabling potentially damaging and self-centred behaviour to be mediated by wisdom and empathy.

Olive works on the meridian system in such a way as to encourage acting and living in a wholly truthful manner. Situations can arise when one 'holds one's tongue' and 'knows one's place'. Olive helps to balance one's needs with the needs of others in a more constructive and fair manner.

It is able to allow a positive flow of emotional energy so that it becomes possible to regain a personal sense of freedom and self-determination. It prevents a build-up of pent up emotion by releasing and expressing it truthfully in a natural and easy manner - rather than with explosive anger. Energy releases those knots of controlled passion, indignation and sense of unfairness so a person can become their own master again without the need to reject the established pattern of relationships with others.

All the chakras are deeply energised, which strengthens the sense of self. Courage and motivation increase to develop practical, down to earth solutions. There is an ability to heal issues of self-worth and sense of value. Problems often arise from a false sense of inferiority or an egotistical altruism, both of which unbalance a proper perspective of how and why one acts as one does. Whenever there is doubt about one's ability to get better, olive brings a positive and soothing energy that can help all forms of illness.

Partly because of its activating solar qualities and also because olive is so good at clearing away the limiting vision things can be seen much more clearly for their own true nature.

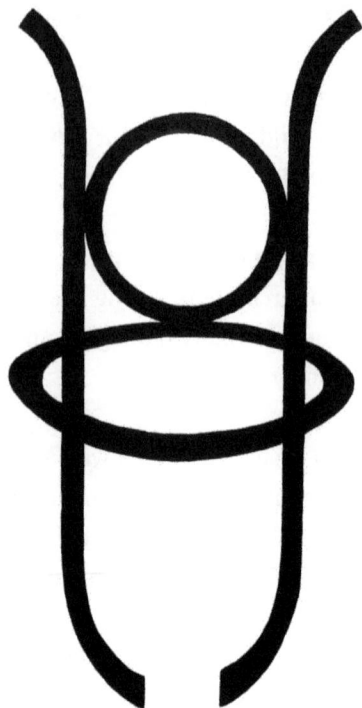

Osier *(Salix viminalis)*

Keywords: spiritual void

Colour: gold

Chakras: 2, 3

Mantra: CHAA   J' FAA   CHAA

Note Sequence:
Ab Ab C A   *C * Eb *F   C* Eb* F * Ab Ab C A
(second section: three notes lower octave, next three upper octave)

Colour Sequence: orange - white

Osier *(Salix viminalis)*

The osier is a member of the willow family that is usually a many-stemmed shrub from 10 - 30ft (3-6m). It is regularly coppiced to create fast-growing shoots or 'withies' used in basket weaving. It can be easily recognised in summer from its very long blade-like leaves, dark green on top and silvery undersides. The leaf edges are toothless and rolled in slightly. The flowers are borne separately as 'pussy willows'.

This essence can be used when there is a need to accept and let go. It will relax the mind and let a deeper wisdom well up.

Osier strengthens the solar plexus chakra, particularly when it seems that a void lies behind existence and everything appears shallow and meaningless. This apparent blackness can be, in reality, an actual experience of the unrevealed, hidden or unmanifest levels of creation which has to be understood for what it is: the underlying vibration of all life.

Osier gives a more balanced approach to one's relationship with others, neither being too forceful or overbearing nor too willing to accept others points of view. A broader understanding of concepts and experiences helps this approach. More energy can be given to personal beliefs so that it isn't felt necessary to indoctrinate others or to get your own way, ignoring the opinion of others.

At the mental level flexibility and creativity are encouraged in the concepts and ideas one holds and osier helps to acquire the wisdom enabling the individual to access and use the fundamental energy of the universe and the wisdom to use personal power correctly.

Signature: Being 'cut down' is no disadvantage for the osier's vitality as then it simply makes more rapid, more flexible and useful shoots. Lack becomes the means to expand.

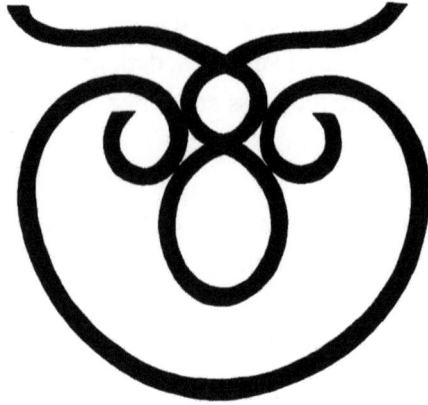

Pear *(Pyrus communis)*

Keyword: serenity

Colour: yellow

Chakra: 3

Mantra: DAY SHIH SHIH DAY

Note Sequence: G F B *Bb *G *F *G *E *D *D

Colour Sequence: pink - yellow - orange - lime green

Pear *(Pyrus communis)*

The native pear, *Pyrus cordata*, is extremely rare existing only around the area of Plymouth, Devon, where it was identified as a separate species at the end of the last century. The common pear is most probably a naturalised tree originating from hybrids in southern Europe.

It is often planted in gardens and parks as well as farmland and orchards. In winter pear is a dark, tall and sparsely branched tree resembling a thorn in many ways.

In April, pear produces white flowers as the leaves emerge. Wild varieties sucker freely and produce small, very gritty fruit. Like apple it can be frequently found along roadsides and footpaths. The tree can reach 50 ft. (15m).

Pear calms fears and brings clarity of mind, increasing the sense of peace and joy. It will help to clear and re-energise the nervous system after it has been blocked by the effects of past-life experiences or powerful belief systems. This encourages a sense of ease and relaxation throughout.

The Gallbladder meridian is cleansed which increases the sense of serenity and happiness. There is a clarity, simplicity, confidence and inner calm: happy to be who one is.

The solar plexus chakra is involved increasing enthusiasm, activation and motivation for physical activity.

At its finest level pear brings a deep peace, an unimpeded flow of communication, a frictionless flow.

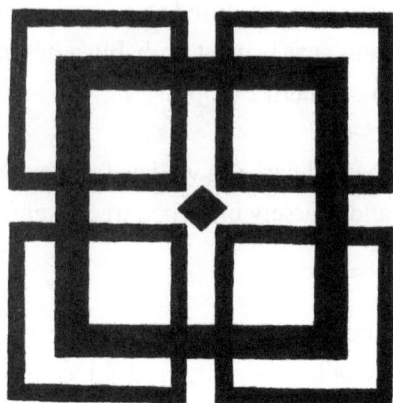

Persian Ironwood *(Parrotia persica)*

Keyword: alienation

Colour: red

Chakra: 1

Mantra: DAA SH. T' HRRIY

Note sequence: G

Colour sequence: violet

Persian Ironwood *(Parrotia persica)*

Persian ironwood is a small native tree of the Caucasus mountains and northern Iran. Persian ironwood is the only member of its genus, though it has features similar to the witch-hazel family. It flowers early in the year, usually January, producing dense clusters of red stamens upon the branches. It is planted as an ornamental for its plane-like bark, autumn foliage of golden-crimson red and the early show of flowers. The wood is so hard as to be unworkable.

Persian ironwood is essentially grounding, earthing and energising in its functions. The essence increases the sense of security and emotional stability, especially when dealing with strong drives and emotions.

There is a greater recognition and understanding of one's intuitive faculties and, as a result, an increased sense of peace and joy as the mental functions become more integrated. At an emotional level, the energising influence enables a greater expression of harmony, love and non-aggression. After all, negative emotions and reactions arise from fears that have their basis in self-doubt and insecurity. When one knows that one is invincible there can be no enemy and no fear.

On very fine levels of energy this tree helps to link to the super-consciousness of the planetary energies as a whole. With this link comes a strong sense of being connected, a new sense of self, and an influx of joy and happiness. It is deeply energising and as such it will tend to activate self-healing processes. As the energies of Persian ironwood ground, the energies of the future into the present, were genetic changes likely to be of use to the individual, this essence might help initiate the process.

 Where there is chronic energy drain and with those who are too 'open' to subtle vibrations causing emotional or physical imbalance, this tree works well. It has also been used to great effect to help those recovering from involvement in natural disasters, such as earthquakes. It helps re-establish confidence in the solidity of the planet.

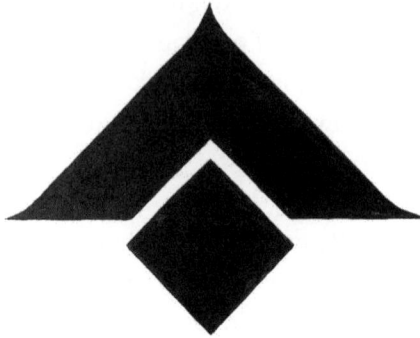

Pittospora, Kohuhu *(Pittosporum tenuifolium)*

Keywords: in two minds

Colours: yellow, violet

Chakra: 3

Mantra: K. G. G. G.
(No vowel sounds nor aspirates, just plosives at the back of the palette whilst breath is held).

Note Sequence: F# G Ab Ab

Colour Sequence: pink

Pittospora, Kohuhu *(Pittosporum tenuifolium)*

This tree is native to the forests between the mountains and the sea of New Zealand's coastline. It can be found in Britain where the winters are mild. Pittospora can grow to 33ft (10m) in a neat, compact, broadly columnar form. The leaves are evergreen with glossy surfaces and a characteristic pronounced wavy margin. It flowers in late spring with small waxy, fragrant deep red-purple petals and bright yellow anthers. Except on the variegated varieties, the flowers can be inconspicuous from a distance.

Pittospora brings clarity of perception and clarity of mind. It gives the ability to see the truth from a broader viewpoint and to act on it in an orderly, organised way.

When one is 'in two minds' and unable to determine where loyalties lie, this essence helps to clarify how we really feel. This releases pressure from the Kidney meridian and also balances the spiritual body.

The clarity and creativity at the finer levels of the self helps to relax anxieties, over-seriousness and lack of humour.

With the new, clearer perspective it is easier to explore what one is really about at a core level. This increases the sense of purpose, mental peace and encourages a truly individual way to be alive.

Signature: The red/purple and yellow flowers suggest the balance of energy between the head(purple) and gut (yellow) levels of reaction. The flowers sit close to the leaf axils, between leaf and stem, and therefore are between two different forms of expression. Just as the tree itself grows in the area between mountains and sea. Hesitancy is suggested by the strongly wavy leaf edges.

Comment: Pittospora is quite a common garden and park tree in the South West of England as the climate tends towards milder winters. It can also be found in Ireland and southern England.

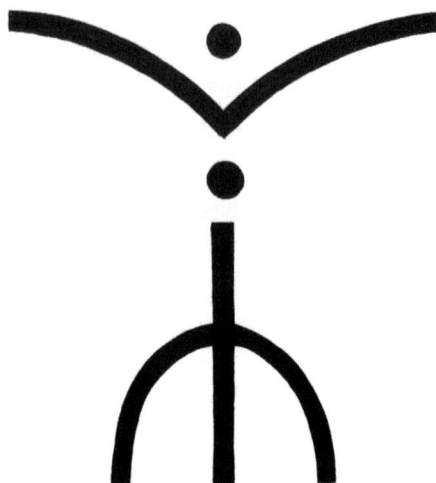

Plane Tree *(Platanus x acerifolia)*

Keywords: fine judgement

Colour: yellow

Chakra: 3

Mantra: NI YO TIE YO

Note sequence: G# Db *Bb *F#

Colour sequence: green - orange - blue - yellow

Plane Tree *(Platanus x acerifolia)*

The Oriental plane (*Platanus orientalis*) is a massive tree that can grow to many thousands of years old. It has a huge, low bole sending out large branches that often rest upon the ground before swinging upwards again. The commonest variety of plane seen is the London plane, a hybrid between the oriental plane and American plane. This is a familiar tree in towns and cities (hence its name) because it survives pollution very well in poor soils. It is, nonetheless, a large forest tree.

Plane tree encourages fine judgement - the ability to discern the truth of a situation. This justice, wisdom and calm clarity derives from a deep tuning into the nature of things. Plane helps to develop a mental structure that is able to cope with the flow of intuition and information.

The essence has a beneficial effect on the Small Intestine meridian preventing too much introspection or dwelling on sadness. It can be useful for those who are prone to over-analyse and who are subject to fits of melancholy. The Gallbladder meridian is also strengthened and this can create a state of detachment where a broader viewpoint can be seen. Again, a peacefulness replaces anxiety and intellectual or organisational over-analysis.

The mental body is relaxed and becomes more open to deeper perceptions and meditative states. Plane tree creates a calm, detached space in which to grow. The ability of the tree to respond positively to outside influences (withstanding pollution, heavy pruning etc.), implies detachment and the ability to let go and see the larger perspective.

Plane trees have a long history of being venerated for their great size and age. It is said that the Persian emperor Darius halted on one of his campaigns to honour a plane tree with sumptuous offerings. Oriental planes, because they are so large and more sensitive to cool weather are less often planted than the vigorous, tough hybrid.

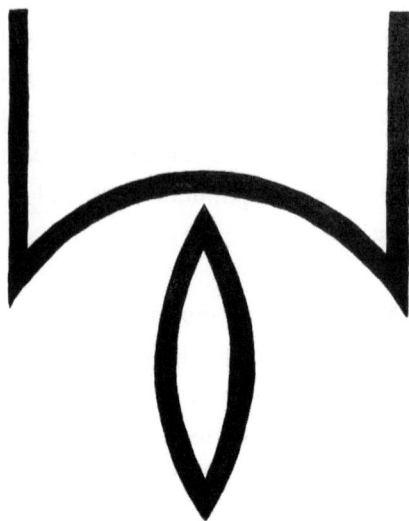

Plum *(Prunus domestica)*

Keyword: empowerment

Colour: magenta

Chakras: 1, 4

Mantra: DAA SHUT

Note sequence: G Db G A

Colour sequence: pink - rainbow - pink

Plum *(Prunus domestica)*

The plum is a common garden and orchard tree. Originally all plums were cultivated in the Middle East by crossing parents of different species. The plum, like its small-fruited varieties the damson and greengage, developed from crosses between the blackthorn and cherry plum. Plum flowers in April and May producing a white, five-petalled blossom that sprinkles the black branches just as the leaves are opening.

For such a small, domestic tree the plum spirit carries great healing power. The energy of plum is the transformation and transmutation of physical activity and material existence by healing, transcendent love. It can access the knowledge and understanding of creation through healing love and the desire to go beyond established boundaries.

There is a sense of freedom and space to achieve the perfect flow of information, communication and peace. It gives the space and freedom to establish peace.

Fears are easier dealt with through understanding their causes and through a clearer use of the intellect - the creative aspect of the rational mind.

The Triple Warmer and Central meridians are supported, helping to counter the innervating emotions of shame and loneliness. There is a clearer understanding of one's place in the universe and an increased awareness of the relationship to all created things, as well as a better ability to express what the heart feels and to experience bliss.

The throat chakra is energised strengthening the sense of personal power, allowing one to accept things as they are and help to bring about practical solutions. The root chakra is also allowed to play a greater part in practical, everyday decision-making, particularly giving access to the instincts.

Although a great deal of spiritual energy is brought in with the plum essence it is directed towards dynamic and practical ends.

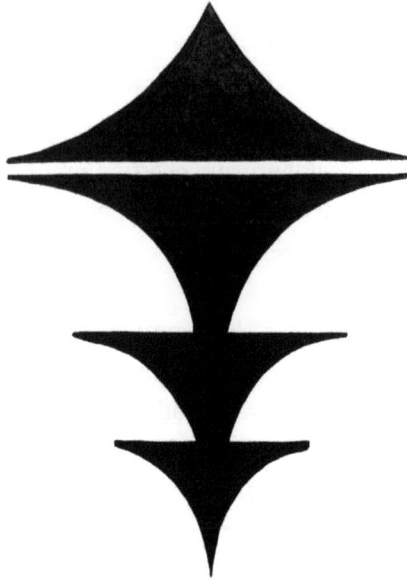

Privet *(Ligustrum vulgare, Ligustrum ovalifolium)*

Keywords: old wounds

Colour: orange

Chakra: 2

Mantra: JOWE DOUGH JUH

Note Sequence: *F *A *A# *G *F

Colour Sequence: black - gold - pink - indigo - black

Privet *(Ligustrum vulgare, Ligustrum ovalifolium)*

Privet is best known as a hedging plant and this species used is *Ligustrum ovalifolium* introduced from Japan in the 1840's to largely replace the native species, *Ligustrum vulgare*. Both plants are similar in form and habit except the native species has smaller leaves and flowers and does not retain its leaves in winter like the Japanese variety. Wild privet can be found in hedgerows and woods easily distinguishable by its smaller scale. The flowers form shiny black berries in autumn, once used in dyeing.

Privet works primarily at the level of the subtle bodies, though there is a slight energising of the meridian system. The main areas it affects are the emotional, astral and causal bodies - that is, the levels of feeling and emotion; the personality and ego; and the collective awareness and past-life influences. There is an increase in energy and life-force in the emotional body that helps the acceptance of growth and change. The astral body is helped to recognise the need to release blocks caused by the physical trauma in this or other lifetimes.

Privet is not particularly effective at emotional levels. It has more focus on structural patterns of programming, and is indicated whenever there is a need to release shock from within the subtle bodies. A harmonious vibration is created that helps to heal and balance the subtle anatomy.

The emotional body very often deals with the individual's reaction to both itself and others. With this is brought into a finer balance with the astral body and the causal body, it becomes clearer what behaviour patterns are simply echoes from distant encounters - a reliving of past dramas. Once this is realised it becomes easier to disengage the automatic responses and see the situation from the present viewpoint. Such rebalancing will also help to put the individual at ease where they may feel out of place.

The privet can be trimmed, shaped and cut throughout the year without harm. It reminds us that wounds and restrictions need not damage us permanently and that recovery is always possible.

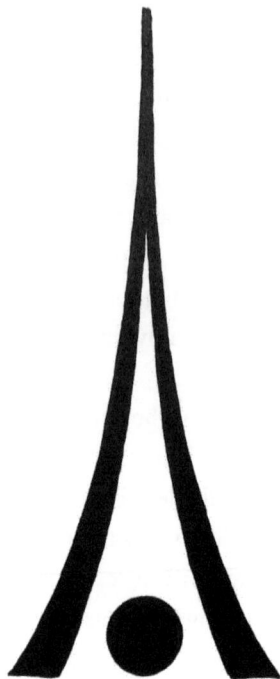

Red Chestnut *(Aesculus x carnea)*

Keywords: fear for others

Colours: red, violet

Chakra: 1

Mantra: BEE TIE

Note sequence: Db E G D

Colour sequence: blue - yellow - blue - green

Red Chestnut *(Aesculus x carnea)*

The red chestnut is a hybrid between the horse chestnut and the red buckeye from North America. It is thought to have originated in Germany and was available in the 1820's. Although a hybrid, it is fertile and breeds true, although most trees are grafted onto the more robust horse chestnut. It is a lighter, much smaller tree reaching a height of 22m (65ft) and is not as long-lived. The leaves are smaller, darker and less splayed than horse chestnut. The spikes of flowers are pink or dark red and appear in May and June.

With red chestnut comes a feeling of security and protection at a very deep level of being. There is a peace and detachment from emotional issues to do with expectancy and hope. This encourages the ability to live in the present rather than with the possibilities of futures.

All the subtle bodies are brought into balance where fears and needs are countered by the awareness of joy and happiness. This arises because the sense of underlying security allows one to deal with and balance up fears and anxieties.

Communication with others is made stronger and without the stabilising balance this essence brings, such close links might upset personal equilibrium and boundaries.

There is a greater balance between the mind and the imagination. This again, helps to resolve fears and phobias caused by experiences in the past.

There is an ability to manifest, or increase the possibility of manifestation, of what one thinks. It is therefore useful that red chestnut encourages a balanced positive view and breaks the hold of self-fulfilling worry.

Signature: The red candles suggest stability and strength of action carrying strong emotions effortlessly with the ability to discard or transform them where appropriate.

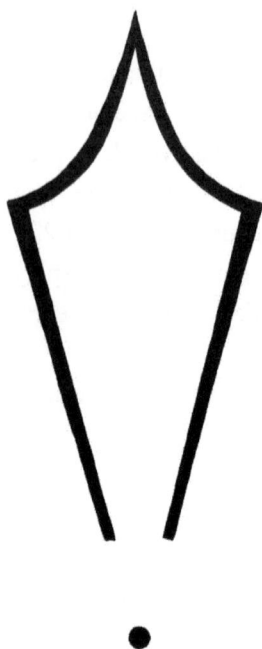

Red Oak *(Quercus rubra)*

Keywords: practical support

Colour: red, violet

Chakra: 1

Mantra: TAY K'HOO PAA KAA GHEY AAA

Note Sequence: B A F F Eb Eb Eb D C

Colour Sequence: white - turquoise - magenta - green - turquoise

Red Oak *(Quercus rubra)*

The red oak is one of the largest deciduous trees in eastern North America. Mature trees grow to 90ft. (27m) with a girth of six to nine feet. The seedlings are the fastest growing of all the oaks – between 7-10ft.(3m) in five years. The leaves are characteristically oak-shaped but with sharp-pointed tips turning a red-orange brown in autumn.

The catkins appear with the bright yellow new leaves and when fertilised the fruit forms acorns that take two years to ripen. The first recorded tree in England is in 1739, though here it rarely lives above 200 years.

The quality of red oak is energising and practical for the mind. It encourages exploration of practical or physical techniques with which to expand self-awareness, such as hatha yoga, Chi Kung and so on.

Red oak energy can increase the amount of energy. The root chakra becomes more closely aligned to the energies of nature. There can be a deeper attachment to the Earth and a deep knowing about one's place and function. This is the nature of the instinctive, right-acting body personality that gives the feeling of what is right to be and do.

The solar plexus chakra is cleared of self-doubt and false self-concepts and is helped to speed the healing of all self-issues.

At the finest level, red oak emphasises the awareness of the individual as a being that is loving and constantly loved. It can find practical outlets for the yearning towards Unity. It will help with the lesson of learning to let go of what is dearest, so that one can be given everything in return.

Signature: The strong earthy-red colouration of the autumn leaves that remain on the tree for many winter months.

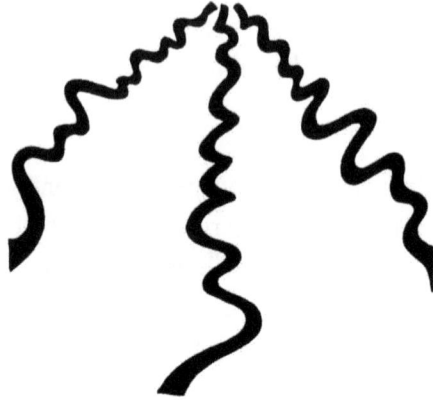

Robinia (Locust Tree, Black Locust, Yellow Locust, False Locust, False Acacia) *(Robinia pseudoacacia)*

Keyword: awakening

Colour: white

Chakra: 5

Mantra: B'HRRUH   HIGH. B'RRUH HIGH. B'RRUH HIGH.

Note Sequence: D D C D E C# C

Colour Sequence: pink - white - gold - green - pink

Robinia (Locust Tree, Black Locust, Yellow Locust, False Locust, False Acacia) *(Robinia pseudoacacia)*

The robinia is an American tree native to the south-eastern States of the US where it can be found in woods and thickets in the Allegheny Mountains and the Middle Mississippi Valley. When the weather is warm enough, robinia flowers in midsummer with cascades of fragrant, white, pea-like flowers. When fertilised these flowers form dark brown seed pods, which originally reminded the American settlers of the locust beans, or carob, native to the deserts of the eastern Mediterranean. This tree and its essence are cooling and calming. It allows the mind to flow in imaginative ways that inspire and create peace rather than, for example, becoming locked in fearful anxieties about future outcomes. A positivity and relaxation help the flow of energy through the body.

When there is some disparity between hopes, wishes, dreams and the actual reality of the situation, robinia helps to bring a new clarity. Locked into imagination people can become isolated and withdrawn from those around them. There is a general enlivening effect based around the throat chakra making it possible to really communicate one's own ideas and concepts and simply to be able to express joyfulness. This subduing of fears and anxieties, focusing more on positive values gives a chance for a better understanding of situations, better memory and clearer intellectual capacity. It creates a cleansing and purification of the mind, a clearing away of old emotional cobwebs.

There is an increase of balance and peace, an ability to take in a larger, less individualised viewpoint, to be able to understand things from a universal perspective where evolutionary forces and the very nature of matter and awareness expand and flow in order to experience and relate in new ways. Robinia clears the mental and emotional clutter created by looking too closely at the details and allows us to get a spacious panorama, to take a deep calming breath, to see that things are flowing and that joy can be had by being real and paying attention to what is going on now. Robinia helps to create the opportunity to expand into the universe a little more effectively.

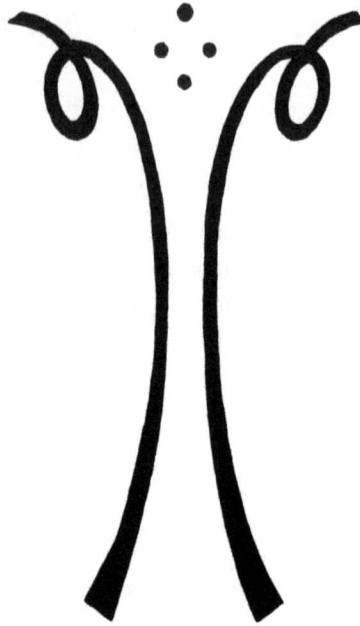

Rowan *(Sorbus aucuparia)*

Keyword: nature

Colour: green, violet

Chakra: 7

Mantra: AY NOO AY

Note sequence: G F F G *F *C#

Colour sequence: red - yellow - blue sparkled with white

Rowan *(Sorbus aucuparia)*

The rowan, also known as the mountain ash, grows at a higher altitude than any other native British tree. In the north, its autumn foliage is the brightest of reds, though further south they fall early.

Rowan enhances the ability to tune into the energies of nature. This is because it encourages focus and discipline and a clearing of perception that allows breakthroughs in awareness in order to contact deeper levels of universal consciousness. This is balanced with the ability to ground information and communication in an integrated and supportive manner.

Rowan helps to overcome illusions and encourage realistic spiritual aims and great creativity. The essence will even foster greater co-creativity as the limited self becomes submerged in its greater nature. The Large Intestine meridian is stimulated helping to calm the emotions and overcome feelings of separation. Letting go and forgiving fears can be uncovered and dissolved.

The heart chakra is filled with a nurturing serenity whilst the crown chakra is enabled to solve emotional blocks and re-configure awareness in a larger, more spacious and supportive environment. The higher chakra, the tenth, is brought to a state of purity, openness, expansion and emptiness, where the universal can easily flow in to the individual.

The subtle bodies are energised though the effects tend to be practical: there can be an improvement in memory and a quietening down of over-excited thought processes. Memory recall is stimulated as is the ability to communicate with deep intuitive levels, cleansing trauma and bringing harmony.

There is an increase in satisfaction and happiness with more space to think and identify needs. The quality of opening up awareness to the universe means that rowan creates a connection to the 'fixed stars', very distant objects, which brings a deeper understanding of the cosmos and the ability to recognise and make use of that energy in a positive, creative way.

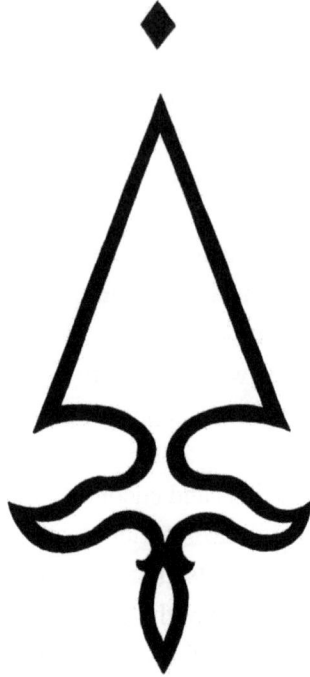

Scots Pine *(Pinus sylvestris)*

Keyword: insight

Colour: green, indigo

Chakra: 6

Mantra: MA-FRRUK T. DAA VA

Note sequence: G A C*

Colour sequence: red - magenta

Scots Pine *(Pinus sylvestris)*

The Scots pine is a pioneer tree that survives well on poor or sandy soil. There are many different forms of Scots pine but those most planted are the tall, straight forms. Although native in the Scottish Highlands, Scots pine was only re-introduced into England around 1660. Scots pine flowers in May and June producing huge amounts of pollen (second only to elm).

The activity of Scots pine focuses on the upper parts of the body. At a physical level the essence can help create calm and relaxation in the chest areas, both relaxing and clearing the lungs, easing breathing and reducing stress from the heart.

It is a cleansing, clearing energy that can help release blockages anywhere in the system. Boundaries are both repaired and maintained, so that individual integrity is enhanced without blocking out energy or information from other sources.

As the boundaries become more secure the heart is opened and calmed and the brow chakra can become greatly energised. This enables a clearer perception of fine levels of energy such as auric and clairvoyant sight. The perception of nature and the kingdoms of nature, especially nature spirits, are made more accessible. But clarity of the brow chakra also functions at the mundane, or anyway less spectacular, levels of seeing. Thus there is a clarity of understanding - seeing at every level, and this means that meditative states are easier to maintain and tend to be more profound. Scots pine brings a penetrating insight and allows a balanced growth of individual gifts. It increases tenacity and patience with the ability to see the broader aspects of good and bad. With this, too, comes forgiveness.

Scots pine effectively grounds excess energy and ensures a practical development of this mental clarity, avoiding a top-heavy, energetic build-up in the body. Dr Edward Bach used a boiled preparation of both male and female flowers to clear guilt, the sense of blame and the failure to live up to one's expectations.

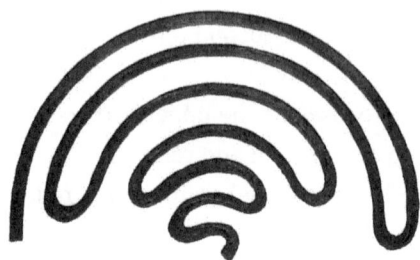

Sea Buckthorn *(Hippophae rhamnoides)*

Keyword: pioneer

Colour: indigo

Chakra: 6

Mantra: VOH SAY JAI JAY SAY

Note Sequence: C C B *G *G

Colour Sequence: white - green - yellow - white..(repeating)

Sea Buckthorn *(Hippophae rhamnoides)*

Sea buckthorn was one of the pioneer species that re-colonised Britain after the last Ice Age. Sea buckthorn is a thorny, low-growing shrub, not usually more than 10ft (3m) in height, except when sheltered from the wind. Female plants bear bright orange berries in great numbers that remain all winter on the branches. These berries have traditionally been made into jelly and are rich in vitamins and minerals.

The clearing away of confusing clouds of emotion is the key to sea buckthorn's actions. It brings clarity of mind and a certain detachment. We can learn better to keep at an appropriate distance from others and remain in a calm, balanced state. Emotionally this can help with issues to do with pride, power-hunting or grasping attitudes - where we seek to impose ourselves onto others and to balance the opposite tendency to remain haughty or aloof by encouraging the ability to communicate feelings and wishes.

This re-balancing will benefit the Gallbladder meridian if suffering from the effects of pride or haughtiness. The Lung meridian is balanced with a more creative way of escaping from the established, unsuccessful, modes of communication with others.

With the essence of sea buckthorn spiritual energies have access to the physical levels of the body, especially by way of the solar plexus and sacral chakras. In this way, spiritual energies integrate with the physical to make it a real, powerful force. The world and the spirit are more easily experienced as inseparable, (which in truth they are). This allows a powerful, personal energy base for developing skills and achieving goals.

In spiritual practices, sea buckthorn brings a quiet mind. It subdues mental processes or creates a detachment from mental processes - including memories and belief systems. Because calm is experienced it is more possible to receive new information. This process favours listening instead of analysing. The use of mantra may also be enhanced with this essence.

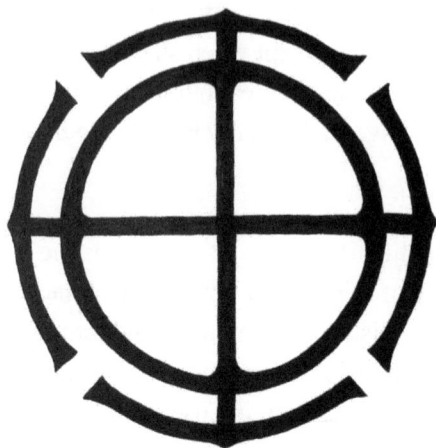

Sequoia *(Sequoia sempervirens)*

Keyword: anchor

Colour: green

Chakra: 4

Mantra: TAA TER SHUSHAA KOOK A

Note sequence: C# C F# G Eb C# C

Colour sequence:
  yellow - red - turquoise - blue - turquoise - gold - red - green

Sequoia *(Sequoia sempervirens)*

Of the three species of redwood, the coast redwood, also called the coastal redwood and California redwood, is the tallest tree on the planet. It can grow up to 380 ft (116 m) and can live for 1,500 years or more. It is thought to be a very ancient hybrid of the two other redwoods, the giant redwood and the dawn redwood. Its natural range is limited to the sheltered valleys of northern California and coastal Oregon, where it thrives on poor soils in conditions of high rainfall and moisture laden fogs.

The sequoia has a narrow, conical crown with slightly drooping branches, making it quite easy to distinguish from the heavy domed profile of giant redwood. It has small, thin spiny leaves with flowers at the end of new growth that resembles the cypresses. The bark is very thick, soft and fire-resistant.

Sequoia brings balance to the whole personality, with a focus on personal space and a sense of belonging. It helps to anchor the self into the reality of physical existence, whilst allowing a flow of life-giving energies from subtle levels.

Sequoia brings calm and a quiet acceptance to stressful situations, with a clarity that encourages positive creative solutions to problems. This flow of energy is expressed through all the qualities of the tree. It encourages personal expression as a means to be honest and fulfilled with our lives. It helps to unblock rigidities that prevent us from enjoying experience, and releases stresses from the past that prevent us from moving on.

The throat chakra is energised to be able to communicate what we feel in a calm and eloquent manner. Calm increases in the mind and there is a quiet confidence in spiritual experiences. There is a reduction in habitual anxiety and in fear of the unknown. Intuition and inspiration are easier to access and the mind becomes less prone to imaginative interpretation of events.

A constant cleansing flow of energy between all levels of existence is what the sequoia manifests in its great, silent presence.

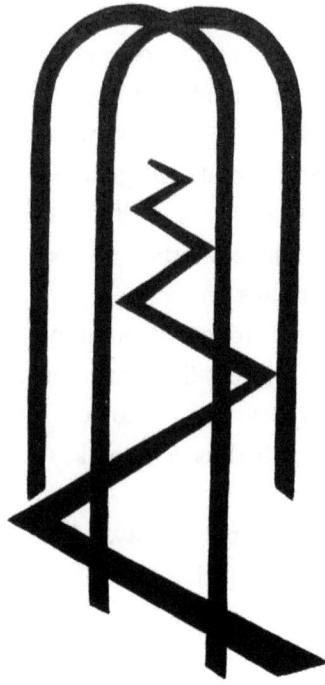

Silver Birch *(Betula pendula)*

Keyword: beauty

Colour: pink

Chakra: 4

Mantra: KOO SHOW TIE PAA

Note sequence: G G F Eb G Eb F

Colour sequence: magenta - gold - indigo - white with blue shimmers

Silver Birch *(Betula pendula)*

The two native birches, the silver birch *(Betula pendula),* and the downy birch *(Betula pubescens),* occupy different environmental niches and have distinct forms although cross-breeding occurs between them. Energetically they bring very similar energies as expressed through the focus of the land.

The spirit of birch brings the ability to experience beauty and calmness. The name of the tree derives from the Indo-European root **bharg* which means bright, shining, white. The experience of beauty is more than a simple appreciation of form: it is an acknowledgement and realisation that everything that is, rejoices in its own nature, its own life - that simply being is sufficient to create endless joy within oneself. Beauty is the acknowledgement of this simple goodness of being, both in oneself and in others.Without the awareness of beauty there can be only separation and division.

Encouraging this quality birch helps to ease harsh judgements of the self and of others. It can give the ability to understand and accept other people's views without criticism. Supporting individuality and nurturing life feed one's surroundings and reflects back life-supporting energy into oneself.

Harmonious sharing is encouraged. This state then allows the further growth and manifestation of new beginnings and new possibilities for great happiness. Birch will be of use to those who find it difficult to express themselves.

The experience of quiet and deep beauty helps to release old patterns of behaviour. Beauty is the experience of the transcendent within the present, and as such this essence effectively dissolves the rigidity and stubbornness that prevents clarity and flexibility of action and perception.

Signature: Birch is a pioneer tree that provides a fertile environment for many other forms of life. The quality of flexibility and grace is apparent in the form.

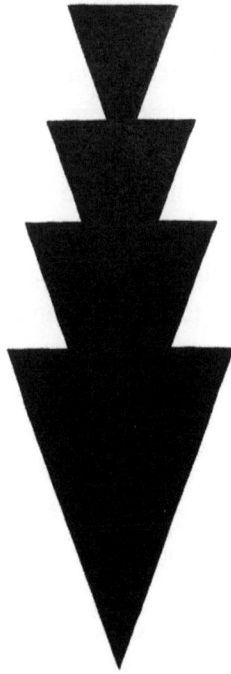

Silver Fir *(Abies alba)*

Keyword: enthroned

Colour: violet

Chakra: 7

Mantra: RAYII HUH HAA J'HAA

Note Sequence: G A E A G D

Colour Sequence: green - red - blue with interlocking white starlight

Silver Fir *(Abies alba)*

The firs have much softer, leathery foliage than the spiky spruces. The silver fir has a smooth light grey-green, neatly cracked bark heavy with resin from which turpentine is made. When given space to grow, the lowest branches can swing upwards to grow parallel to the main trunk. Silver fir is the prominent native forest tree of the Central European mountains and it is the largest fir except for those growing in the American Rockies.

With this tree comes the energy to empower and manifest one's desires with wisdom and skill. It is in essence, deeply protective because it gives practical expression to the individual's true nature. Going in harmony with one's inherent abilities and skills automatically ensures greater safety and success. The Liver meridian is strengthened by this ability to follow the natural flow of energy, accepting the circumstances that arise in life and making changes to accommodate wherever necessary. This ensures that a positive attitude and cheerfulness are easily maintained, which allows for the maximum growth and transformation within the individual life.

Of the chakras, the crown is most activated by this essence. The effect is to firmly root and establish the individual into their universal context. As the root chakra at the base of the spine links us into the Earth's greater energy body, so the crown chakra above the top of the head links us into the universal energy web. Between these two links our energy flows as if within the wires of an electric cable.

With silver fir there is an increase in optimism and positive action. Impetus is given to those activities that bring personal happiness and contentment. Emphasis is given to doing things, to practical solutions and to dynamic expressions of joy in living and enables creative visions to be rooted in practical reality. There is a better ability to achieve personal potential - largely through an increasing fascination in watching the ways that creativity unfolds within the mind and then moves out into the world. This interest in the pathways of manifestation, in how energy moves, grows and changes, also teaches us the skills to maintain the balance within ourselves.

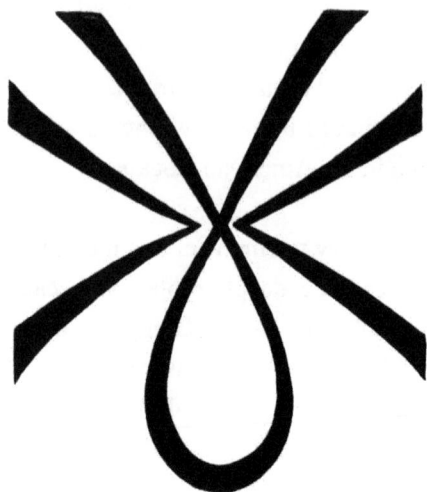

Silver Maple *(Acer saccharinum)*

Keyword: moods

Colours: blue, pink

Chakras: 2, 4

Mantra: TESH YOONOOSH. NOW

Note sequence: A Bb G C# G

Colour sequence: green - yellow - magenta

Silver Maple *(Acer saccharinum)*

Many maples can be found planted throughout Britain for their decorative colours and shapes. Silver maple comes from the eastern coast of North America where it is one of the main sources of sugar and maple syrup extracted from the sap in springtime. In Britain, the sugar content is not high enough for this use, but silver maple is one of the most widely planted as it is hardy (especially in the south of Britain), and grows to 100ft (30m) with an open crown that casts little shade.

Silver maple flowers in early spring with small reddish flowers appearing on the shoots before the leaves open. Silver maple can be easily identified by its rounded, deeply lobed leaves and irregular teeth. The undersides show silver-green in the wind giving the tree a subtle, shifting colouration.

Silver maple essence helps to balance the flow of energy through the body. It is particularly useful for integrating the various meridians into a more balanced flow. Silver maple reduces energy blocks and turbulence, increasing the vitality and life-energy available at any one time.

Where there is a harshness experienced in one's moods, or where there is sensitivity to food substances that results in mood swings, this essence can help the body to restore balance.

Like all maples, silver maple has an energy that increases the experience of stability and sweetness in life.

Signature: The sweet, sugar-rich sap of silver maple : the flow of life-energy and sustenance through the body's subtle channels and circulatory systems. Changing moods: the shifting colours as the leaves are turned in the breeze to reveal the light undersides and then the darker tops of the leaves.

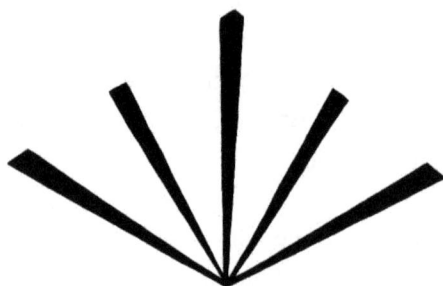

Spindle *(Euonymus europaeus)*

Keyword: self-integration

Colours: white, gold

Chakra: 7

Mantra: HOO P'HAA HOO P'HAA

Sound Sequence: E E F# F# E

Colour Sequence: orange - yellow - red - pink - orange

Spindle *(Euonymus europaeus)*

A small tree growing to 20ft, spindle has a neat, fine form, which although quite common in hedgerows, makes it fairly inconspicuous. Young stems are identifiable by having alternate vertical stripes of green and grey-brown bark. In summer there are a profusion of four-petalled, star-like flowers of greenish white that become unmistakable four-lobed red fruits containing orange seeds in autumn.

There is peace and balance: a communication with deep levels of intuitive mind regarding one's place and direction. Individual nature attunes to the Higher Self allowing self-expression in accord with one's true nature without negative, egotistical feelings of superiority. This helps to remove the tendency to judge others, to be competitive, the need to succeed or be first at every opportunity - a stabilising of Lung meridian functions.

The heart chakra and the solar plexus chakra work together enabling a discernment of a true purpose, a way of life, in which one feels at home and motivated to achieve. The brow chakra is energised for finer levels of perception and communication. The astral body, the integrated personality vehicle, is helped to cleanse the energy patterns of negativity and separation from the personality. A great energising on soul levels.

There is an ability to look at and understand the deepest, darkest, most hidden parts of the self. To understand and accept the Shadow self. The Shadow is that which we have decided is not us, the traits and qualities that have been rejected through every stage of our lives, which are as defining and as much a part of our constructed self-image as those qualities we readily identify with.

To bring light and wisdom into the most hidden levels of existence. Transformation and awareness of what appears negative. Apparent negativity is able to be absorbed and transmuted. Those energies within the self that have been suppressed through fear are relaxed so that stagnant, negative energy can be transformed into life-supporting, dynamic energy.

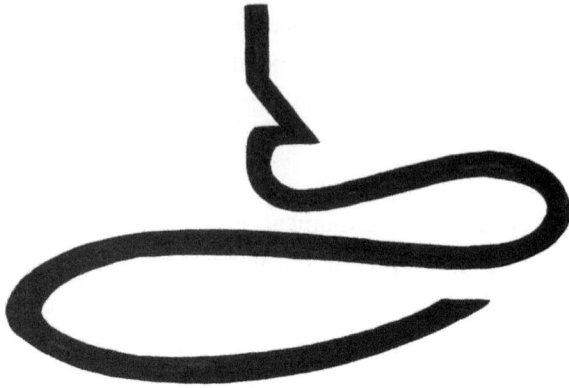

Stag's Horn Sumach *(Rhus typhina)*

Keyword: meditation

Colour: violet

Chakra: 7

Mantra: J'CHO K'LA B'RA

Note sequence: A C* C* Bb F *A A

Colour sequence: green - violet - turquoise

Stag's Horn Sumach *(Rhus typhina)*

Stag's horn sumach is native to meadows, scrub and woodland margins of eastern North America. It may have got its name from the Sumac Indians who were familiar with the tree and its many properties. The stems were used as tobacco pipes and tubes, the fruits eaten and the bark used as a healing astringent and antiseptic. It was brought to Britain in 1629 by John Parkinson.

It is a small tree growing to 26ft (8m) with an open crown and widely spreading habit. It throws up suckers all around the base, though because it can be cut back heavily it is still a common garden tree. The leaves are long with many toothed leaflets. Stag's horn sumach flowers in summer usually with male and female spikes on separate trees, the male a loose cluster of greenish-yellow flowers, the female a tighter spike of rusty red. These ripen into fruit with a sour but edible taste and remain on the furry stems all winter.

The essence of stag's horn sumach has an effect of releasing tension in the area of the throat chakra. At subtle levels too, this tree focuses on the head centres. The brow chakra and related minor chakras are energised, as is the mental body.

It enables the flow of intuition and expression of the Higher Will. This is because it activates the mental body where belief systems, reality models and self-images are held. Sumach initiates a calmness and non-attachment on emotional levels that allows more freedom to access valid supportive actions (hence useful for determining spiritual direction), particularly when in a meditative state.

Stag's horn sumach is an excellent tree to help balance the energies for meditation. It is cooling, stilling the mental and emotional processes and allowing an easier flow of information and energy together with an increased awareness of underlying reality and the ability to perceive harmonious and unifying characteristics of existence.

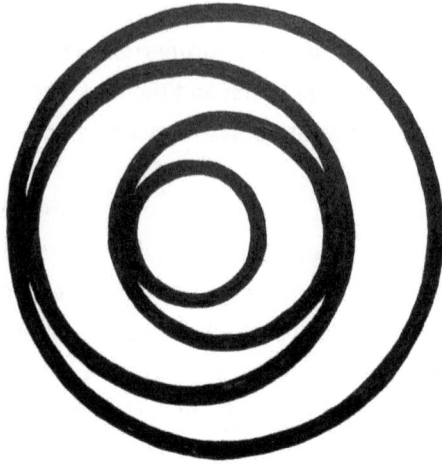

Strawberry Tree *(Arbutus unedo)*

Keyword: quietude

Colours: white, indigo

Chakra: 6

Mantra: KEEN YEAR KOO SHAA. KEEN YEAR KOO SHAA.

Note Sequence: F# D G E A F# F#

Colour Sequence: blue - yellow

Strawberry Tree *(Arbutus unedo)*

This is a small tree growing to 30ft (9m) with a short trunk often laying along the ground and with twisting branches. Its distribution is patchy but is truly native in south-west Ireland where it grows on seaward cliffs. Elsewhere in Britain it grows well in sheltered places, though is usually shrubby. The evergreen leaves are regular, toothed with a white central vein. Strawberry tree flowers in September and October with green-white heather like flowers hanging in loose clusters. The fruit takes two years to ripen, beginning as small green globes, then expanding to yellow and finally red, fleshy spheres. Ripe fruit and flowers can be seen together. The fruit is quite edible though too subtle for some tastes.

Strawberry tree has a focused and specific effect. It primarily stimulate the crown chakra increasing potential for healing and personal spiritual growth. The qualities of the imagination and inspiration are encouraged.

The mind is quietened and cleared. Strawberry tree can almost instantly reduce the levels of mental noise to the merest whisper. It is experienced as a sudden whitening or clearing of thought from the head. This is not calming as such - the emotions are not involved, simply a reduction in noticeable thought processes is allowed.

Transformation occurs through this stillness and silence. As movement and activity dictates all form, it requires a cessation of activity and movement in order to effect change. Ceasing to move allows form to become more fluid and less bound. This can create an opportunity to clear the effects of past actions, habits, and routine thought patterns.

A mature strawberry tree in full autumn sunshine with bright red fruits, yellow orange fruit, milky flowers amid glossy green leaves brings to mind those Otherworldly Celtic trees that bear fruit and flowers simultaneously, or have all kinds (colours) of fruit. Altogether a magical tree that is just about hanging on to very small pockets of habitat throughout Europe, as though the remnants of older times.

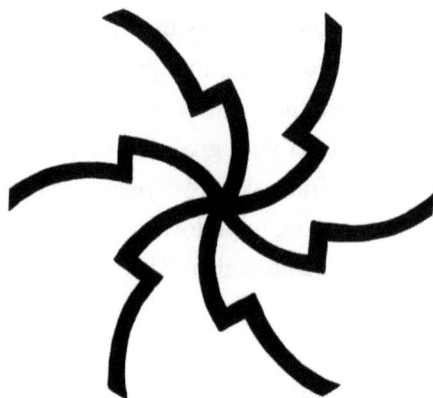

Sweet Chestnut *(Castanea sativa)*

Keywords: the Now

Colour: pink

Chakra: 4

Mantra: DIRREL DOW RAITH

Note Sequence: C# F# C D D C* E E C#

Colour Sequence: magenta - dark green - black - blue - red - magenta

Sweet Chestnut *(Castanea sativa)*

Sweet chestnut, or Spanish chestnut, grows wild in southern Europe, North Africa and the Near East. It is particularly common in Spain. It can grow to 100ft. The larger trees develop a noticeable spiral twist in the bark. Male catkins appear in long yellow tassels in summer at the tips of the branches and the smaller green, rounded female flowers can be found near the leaf bases. The leaves are long, narrow and glossy green with saw-toothed edges. The fruits develop into paired nuts within a green prickly shell.

With sweet chestnut energy there comes an intuitive understanding of underlying harmony and balance. It becomes easier to communicate hidden emotions and feelings in a clear way. This allows deep peace into the heart and emotions.

Central and Heart meridians are balanced and this re-establishes centring, focus and respect for the self. There is a release of stress, shock and trauma that allows creativity to flourish in a way that expresses the individual energy pattern. This can profoundly affect healing and growth on spiritual levels. The brow chakra becomes better able to function, which makes it easier to formulate strategies and find creative ways out of difficult situations.

All the subtle bodies become more integrated and there is an increased confidence in the physical body, improving the sense of well-being. Validation of physical existence in this way helps to remove any sense of guilt and clarifies the personal awareness of right and wrong.

Sweet chestnut helps to release this deep guilt particularly where it focuses on a lack of love for physical existence, physicality itself, strong passions and desires and anything 'earthy'. It can be especially useful for those who feel uncomfortable about physicality as being 'unspiritual'. It encourages the truth that the physical is holy and not a sinful mistake. The essence also helps to bring the ability to accept change on the physical plane and creates a doorway whereby cosmic and universal loving energies can enter the physical system.

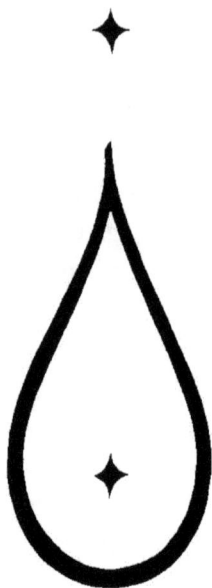

Sycamore *(Acer pseudoplatanus)*

Keywords: lightening up

Colour: yellow

Chakra: 3

Mantra: SH. AW (as in 'shower', 'found')

Note sequence: G C *Bb

Colour sequence: green - orange

Sycamore *(Acer pseudoplatanus)*

The sycamore, great maple or great plane, is the largest of the maple family. It is native to the mountain chains of Europe where it grows in rich, damp soil singly or in groups. The date of its introduction to Britain is not known though sycamore is first mentioned in 1551. Sycamore is a fast-growing tree that spreads rapidly tending to shade out other plants.

There is an increase in the awareness of the sweetness of life, which encourages further growth and fulfilment. All the meridians are strengthened, but particularly the Bladder meridian, encouraging the positive emotional states of peace, harmony, balance and the resolution of conflicts.

The Circulation-Sex meridian also brings the ability to relax, to become more generous and giving and to be able to let go of past issues and events rather than hanging onto them and basing the present moment on past attitudes and outcomes.

The throat chakra, brow and crown chakras are activated. These centres will bring a broader view, clearer insight and a greater ability to make changes that matter. There is thus an overall increase in empowering information and understanding.

Greater acceptance, tolerance and understanding occurs in emotional and mental states. Once this release and relaxation begins it is easier to experience the main energy of the sycamore spirit, which is the activation of the potential to communicate healing energy and to know that one is sustained and protected by the deepest universal levels of love and understanding.

Many people consider sycamore to be little more than a weed, crowding out other, more appropriate native trees. It is true that sycamore makes few niches for other species, yet its fast growth and excellent wood, not to mention the wonderful biomass, would make it a fine forest timber tree for hardwood.

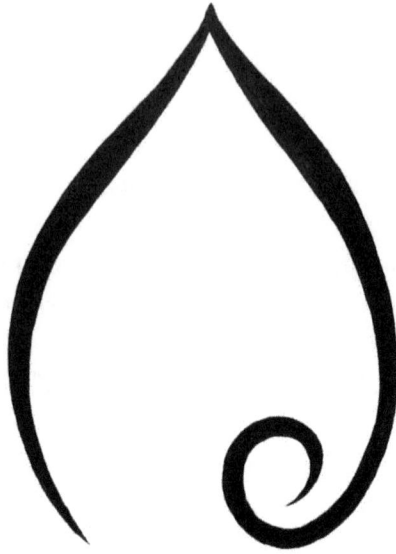

Tamarisk *(Tamarix gallica/anglica)*

Keywords: fire of transformation

Colour: white

Chakras: 2, 3

Mantra: TOO

Note Sequence: Eb G Bb D* Eb G G * F# *E

Colour Sequence: slate blue/grey - blue - red - colour of sunlight on water

Tamarisk *(Tamarix gallica/anglica)*

Familiar on southern coastlines, especially when it bears spikes of pink flowers in summer, tamarisk originates from the Middle East where it was recognised for its medicinal properties. Tamarisk was introduced to Britain as a healing herb in 1582 and has become naturalised in coastal areas where its tolerance to salt and dry climates helps it thrive in harsh conditions. The delicate feathery foliage and mass of flowers have made varieties of tamarisk popular as garden plants. Flowering tamarisk resembles nothing so much as wafts of pink, wind-blown sea foam borne on green feathery waves.

Tamarisk essence is about understanding one's place at the centre of creation. It brings the awareness of one's emergence from the Absolute, and place within the Absolute, even when in the midst of the relative worlds. Because of this knowledge there is total freedom, total flexibility, complete understanding that all is possible. The divine spark leaping from the central sun of Being.

It tunes the energies of the solar plexus chakra into intelligent and evolutionary ways to direct the personal will, life-force, personality and lifestyle. It can be like harnessing for the Higher Self one's chariot of power.
The spiritual body is cleansed and healed, which increases clarity in personal energy on the finest of levels. This will tend to cleanse and transform the ability to manifest and use the finest spiritual energies (the 'ethers'), so that these can be integrated into the net of the energy field. Thus there is the possibility of deep cleansing and the healing of profound shock.

An essence for spiritual direction, freeing up energies for personal expansion and growth. Tamarisk is uplifting and helps shift age-old dross so that the true self can emerge. To paraphrase the Upanishads: "burning the seeds of karma in the furnace of Being".

Signature: Growing by the ocean tamarisk is between two worlds, land and sea. The ocean of possibilities is within its experience and it is adapted to the force that the ocean can display

197

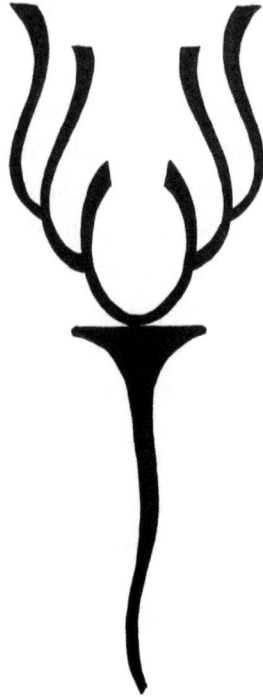

Tree Lichen *(Usnea subfloridana)*

Keyword: wisdom

Colour: violet, white

Chakras: 3, 4

Mantra: KOOCK IN YAA TAY (x3)

Note sequence: D *G# *B C#

Colour sequence: green - yellow

Tree Lichen *(Usnea subfloridana)*

Lichens of various shapes and sizes grow on trees where pollution levels are low and other environmental conditions are suitable. The temperate rainforests of north-west America, for example, and the high-altitude woods of Dartmoor and Wales are home to an abundance of lichen species. Though not a tree itself, the lichen that lives on the branches of trees partake of the ambient energy of their surroundings. Slow growing, living for many years and dwelling in that borderland of definition, neither in contact with the earth yet relying on the rootedness of trees, they consist of two symbiotic plants with distinct healing qualities.

The energy of tree lichen is particularly powerful and its wisdom is profound. The primary energy is purifying and protecting, and indeed it has been said that usnea's prime purpose is to support and protect the life of the trees. It brings the ability to let go of anything no longer needed in order to grow more fully. There comes a greater knowledge and understanding, (particularly on a feeling level), of the cyclical nature of time and events.

An integration of the mental, causal and spiritual bodies brings knowledge of the soul outside time. There is an improved ability to access past knowledge and ancient wisdom. Indeed this freedom from the construct of time and space allows one to communicate with beings beyond the solar system. It brings the ability of going everywhere without going anywhere.

All the chakras can be brought into balance including the minor chakras in the centre of the palms and small chakras in the centre of the ears. A general process of purification and cleansing is encouraged. Tree lichen is an ethereal essence that is rooted in physical existence and the knowledge of the past. It brings a sense of independence and detachment without isolation.

Growing in shade, particularly on the north side of trees, tree lichen has affinity to the Pole Star which itself is the doorway to understanding and experiencing the whole universe. Tree lichen has access to Earth energy indirectly through the tree but lives fully open to cosmic energies.

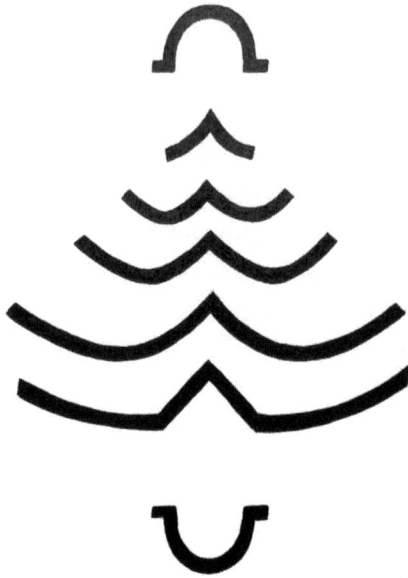

Tree of Heaven *(Ailanthus altissima)*

Keywords: heaven on earth

Colours: red, violet

Chakras: 2, 7

Mantra: D'H.. B.. D'HAY RUH

Note Sequence: G C# *G *D

Colour Sequence: red - blue - gold - black

Tree of Heaven *(Ailanthus altissima)*

The tree of heaven originates from China and was introduced into Britain in 1751. It does well in mild climates and is planted as an ornamental tree in many towns. In very warm climates it seeds and suckers freely. Tree of heaven resembles ash, with opposite leaflets, but is distinguished by a notch on each near the stalk and often there is no terminal leaflet. The leaves open red very late, usually at the end of June, and also fall early. Trees are separately male and female with flowers of greenish-yellow clusters forming large panicles at the end of the shoots. The female flowers ripen to a red-brown winged fruit. Tree of heaven is an open crowned, broadly columnar tree with wriggly branches growing to 65ft (20m).

Tree of heaven gives dynamic, energising spiritual qualities whilst protecting the integrity of the subtle body systems. It energises practical spirituality and practical wisdom.

The crown chakra becomes energised and grounded so that its energy is more easily accessible to other systems of the body. It supplies sufficient energy that this essence will help to break through any blocks at the spiritual level.

Minor chakras at the centre of the forehead help to clarify the understanding of larger truths and ideals, universal concepts and past life viewing. A chakra at the medulla oblongata is stimulated to integrate the experience of bliss onto the physical, thus allowing the experience of the spiritual into the physical.

There is the ability to resolve emotional trauma and obsolete emotional beliefs held in the emotional body. Within the finer levels of personal consciousness there is a greater possibility for the integration and healing of subtle injuries and shock.

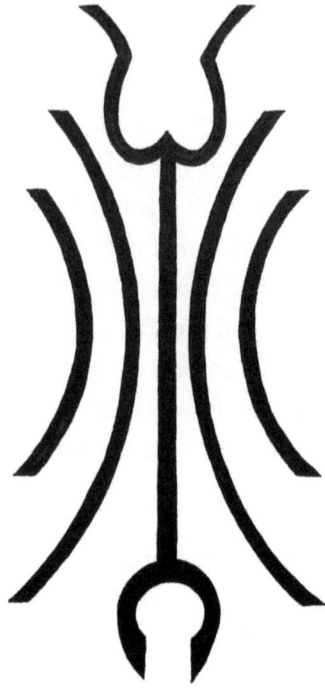

Tulip Tree *(Liridendron tulipifera)*

Keywords: spiritual nourishment

Colours: yellow, blue

Chakra: 2

Mantra: SHA S. HO

Note sequence: *G   C   *E

Colour sequence: turquoise - yellow - green

Tulip Tree *(Liridendron tulipifera)*

The tulip tree, tulip poplar or yellow poplar is native to the eastern United States. It is fast-growing and can reach a height of 50ft in ten or eleven years. It will flower after twenty years and continues to flower for a further two hundred years. It is a tall tree that can grow up to 120ft (37m). It was first planted in Britain in the second half of the 17th century at Fulham. The tree is named for its tulip-like flowers that open greenish-yellow with a blush of orange and pink in mild climates. The leaves are a unique four-lobed shape on long stalks that allow them to flutter like poplar leaves in any breeze.

Tulip tree essence encourages practical outlets for thought processes and wisdom from the Higher Self. There is increased motivation for self-expression.

It balances the Stomach meridian, which brings nourishment at spiritual levels. Where there is spiritual hunger, a gnawing emptiness, tulip tree will bring the means to fulfil personal creativity whilst also bringing increased feelings of connectedness and belonging. The Small Intestine meridian is also affected. There is relief from sorrow and an increase in peace and understanding. This can also strengthen the links to the spirit worlds.

It is possible to remove deep blocks to personal creativity and expression with this essence. Tulip tree will strongly affect the balance of the throat chakra. Artistic abilities will be more likely to manifest and there will generally be an increase in mental creativity and communication skills. The release of long-term stresses encourages greater depths of meditative experiences and an increased clarity and peace. Strong emotional responses, particularly spontaneous reactions, are able to be easier controlled and less volatile in nature.

Signature: This is a tall, narrow tree that flowers from the lowest branches to the top of the crown. Although not conspicuous in colouring the flowers are large and elegant in shape and suggest the flowering of skills at many different levels of awareness.

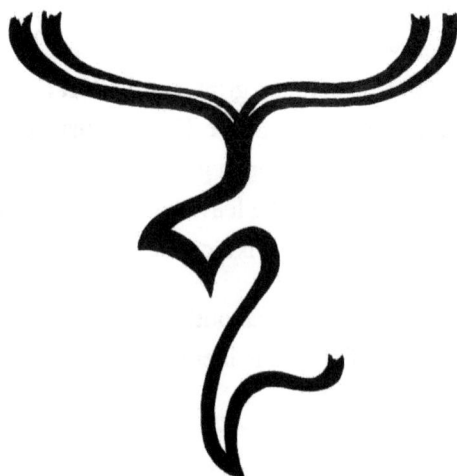

Viburnum *(Viburnum tinus)*

Keyword: reassurance

Colour: pink

Chakra: 4

Mantra: DRRR UNG IH J'HER UB

Note Sequence: F# G G D D E

Colour Sequence: pink - sensation of light (no specific colour, nor white)

Viburnum *(Viburnum tinus)*

Viburnum tinus is native to southern Europe and the Mediterranean. It is a large evergreen shrub or small tree with waxy, white clusters of sweet smelling flowers that appear as long lived clusters in autumn and over winter into springtime, depending on the weather conditions.

The main code of this essence is emotional peace, the flow of peace and an easy communication of feelings. Viburnum helps to find practical ways to establish one's place and feel supported. There is the growth of a balanced assertiveness and an integration and expression of one's own sense of peace and how the world is perceived. This results from a strengthening of the Governing meridian, which dictates the quality of support an individual feels, and the Gallbladder meridian in its aspect of encouraging humility.

Mental activity and individual belief systems are integrated in order to deepen levels of perception and real peace. Inner conflicts will tend to be understood and eased.

At a much finer level, where we initiate the tendencies to act in certain ways, there is a healing of deep trauma. The energy of viburnum is able to initiate extremely deep levels of healing and will help to re-integrate fragmentation caused by near-death experiences and life threatening situations.

Working with the causal and mental bodies viburnum eases any sense of vulnerability, sensitivity, neuroses, feelings of being unhappy or unsettled.

Reassurance and the re-evaluation of past experiences in the light of a broader, more positive outlook is encouraged.

From the underlying connecting energy of all consciousness, there comes a communication from the heart of things.

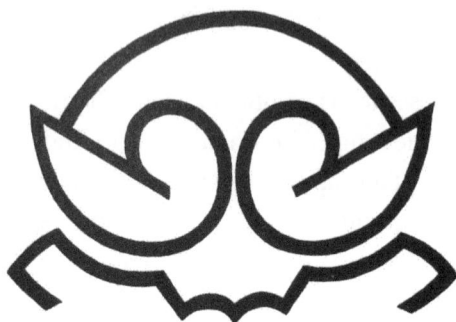

Walnut *(Juglans regia)*

Keyword: liberation

Colour: green

Chakras: 4, 5

Mantra: SHAY SHL' SHAY NOO

Note Sequence: F# G Ab C# Eb C

Colour Sequence: turquoise - red - white - orange - red - white

Walnut *(Juglans regia)*

The natural range of walnut is from Central Asia and China, Iran, Asia Minor, to the Balkans. In Britain it is mostly found in the south and central areas but has been planted as a parkland tree in the north of Scotland. Walnut prefers deep fertile soils and warm summers.

The clear, well-known property and effect of walnut essence is familiar from the Bach Flower Remedies, where it is characterised as a link-breaker. There is a marked cleansing of the Heart meridian, which is linked to the emotional expression of love and forgiveness and their opposites, hate and blame. The clarity that walnut initiates reveals a person's real motivations in life - where one has begun, where one hopes to be going - and this knowledge gives a sense of security. Knowing oneself is really the only way to recognise and combat the influence of other people and other circumstances outside of oneself.

In the Large Intestine meridian, walnut energy creates purification and cleansing. It becomes more possible to let go of things that are no longer appropriate or necessary. This meridian is also affected by the emotions surrounding the concepts of worthiness, goodness and cleanliness. 'Not good enough', 'dirty!', 'bad!', 'unworthy', are all judgements that become lodged in the belief systems whilst still a young child. They limit our potential for growth and personal achievement.

Walnut creates a sense of safety, a self- containment of the sacral chakra that allows a grounding, centring and quietening to establish the fertile ground for personal creativity.

Being less open to unwanted influences, knowing our own qualities, and accepting ourselves, it becomes possible to be really happy just as oneself. Walnut shakes us awake from someone else's dream within which we find we have been living, tells us who we are and lets us fully experience and enjoy our uniqueness.

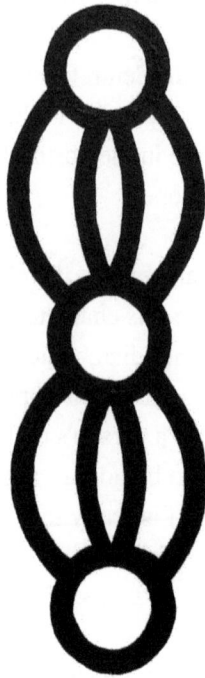

Wayfaring Tree *(Viburnum lantana)*

Keywords: far memory

Colours: green, violet

Chakras: 4, 6

Mantra: T'HOO CHEE S.... T'HRR RRUD HIH

Note Sequence: D *F G *F

Colour Sequence: magenta - magenta centre expanding outwards to turquoise - gold

Wayfaring Tree *(Viburnum lantana)*

Named thus by Gerard in the sixteenth century because of its prevalence along the lanes of southern England, its older name is hoarwithy ('white plant stem'). A small shrub tree, it is easily identified from its strong-looking opposite leaves on short, stout stems. In May and June a dense umbel of white flowers appears on each branch-ending, ripening to shiny black berries. Hoarwithy prefers dry alkaline soils and is rarely found in the North of Britain.

This essence links to specific memories of the place where it is growing. It recognises and calls up similarities of circumstance and patterns that are repeating in the present. Indirectly this can give access to the mechanisms for remembering personal past existences. Wayfaring tree may also help with other temporal sensitivity as in psychic archaeology and psychometry. Working with the tree *in situ* can be very revealing as to a view of times past.

The heart chakra energies are cleared and lightened of emotional burdens such as fear, jealousy, envy etc. There is an ability to focus on choices for life direction and growth.

The etheric body is strengthened, re-establishing its boundaries and independence. This creates a protective space that encourages health of the physical body.

It allows an increased balance of internal energies and polarities that supports information to flow in from other dimensions. Protection against negatively and pollution. Integration with planetary awareness. The essence is supportive of changes in spiritual life.

Signature: found on old paths and uplands-where our ancestors established themselves first. Strong, heart-shaped leaves. Extreme flexibility of stems-even greater than hazel. 'Tying things together'.

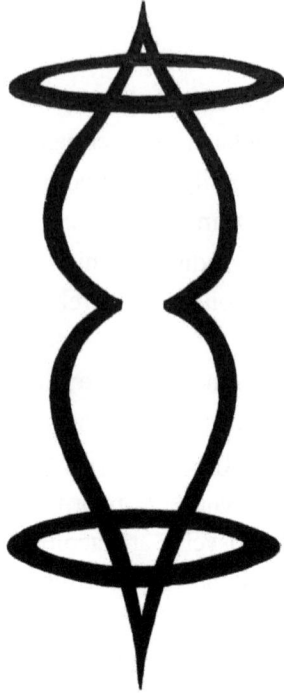

Weeping Willow *(Salix x chrysocoma)*

Keyword: Ego

Colour: gold

Chakra: 3

Mantra: Y RAA TIE

Note sequence: F# Bb C C

Colour sequence: turquoise with green flashes and sparkles of gold

Weeping Willow *(Salix x chrysocoma)*

A tree everybody recognises, weeping willow is a hybrid between Chinese and European parents and grows near rivers and watercourses with other willows and poplars. It was thought to have moved westwards along the Silk Route as woven baskets and crates.

Like most willows, weeping willow has a deep link to the solar energies. Its main focus is the balancing of power. Power can be both life-supporting and life-damaging, like gentle sunlight or the fierce desert sun. Weeping willow helps to balance the extremes of energy. At its finest level it is the spiritual fire, the manifestation of wisdom and beneficial energy to all.

It works with aspects of the Spleen meridian and Lung meridian energy. The essence deals with the negative ego-based states of cynicism and contempt - both of which originate from a false sense of self-righteousness, or at best a failure to accept other people's views as valid.

The emotions and passions are helped to quieten, increasing generosity to others and calms agitated or bad-tempered states.

Weeping willow will help to ameliorate the contempt that arises because one fears that one is perhaps wrong, or that a personal world-view is not unassailable and may, indeed, be invalid. It brings on new creative freedom and the strength to accept to accept another point of view.

The etheric body is given support, particularly to those areas where there is some belief system difficulty with that body part or system. Thus the essence can help to mend the underlying breaches in all-accepting love and compassion that can allow serious physical problems to manifest.

Useful in situations of emotional hurt and sense of loss, it helps re-establish one's true worth and value within creation : equal to all, but superior to nothing.

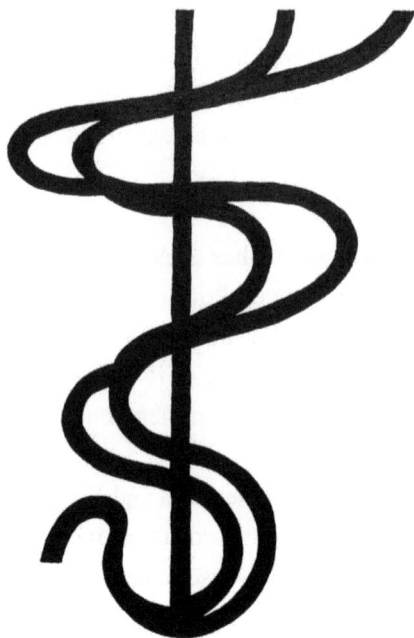

Western Hemlock *(Tsuga heterophylla)*

Keywords: open grace

Colour: white

Chakras: 6, 7

Mantra: OOO PHOO KO

Sound sequence: C# Bb Eb Eb F# Eb

Colour Sequence: yellow - red - magenta

Western Hemlock *(Tsuga heterophylla)*

The hemlocks are a small group of trees similar to spruce, native to North America. They were given this confusing name because the foliage was thought to have the rodent-like smell of *Conium maculatum*, the common umbelliferous hemlock that grows in European hedgerows. Whereas this herb is extremely toxic, the hemlock spruces are quite medicinal.

Where there is the confusion of too many options, the potential of too many possible outcomes, western hemlock will reduce the noise so that what is really there can be clearly seen and be distinguished from speculation. Equally, when there seems to be an absence of options, where nothing seems to be achievable, the essence can sharpen the insight to discover new possibilities. The energy is cleansing, clearing, quietening and focusing.

The crown chakra is brought into this process with an influx of serenity. This clear state of calm awareness also benefits the whole of the energies of the body, helping to identify and remove energy intrusions that do not belong.

An aspect of the Heart chakra concerned with vengeance and forgiveness is activated with this tree energy. These feelings have to do with holding onto pain and letting go of pain. The pretence of forgiveness where none really exists, or giving in to the will of others for the sake of reducing conflict, is replaced with a real relaxation of acceptance - neither ignoring the hurt nor seeking vengeance for wrongs. The cleansing energy of western hemlock allows new beginnings to be simply that: starting with a clean sheet.

Aggravation and anxiety of the mind is calmed and peace increases. It becomes easier to understand the opposite viewpoint to the view that one holds true, and so the roots of selfish conflict can be more easily avoided. Acceptance and relaxation into an honest, open state quietens the mind and enables deeper spiritual insight to enter into more meditative states.

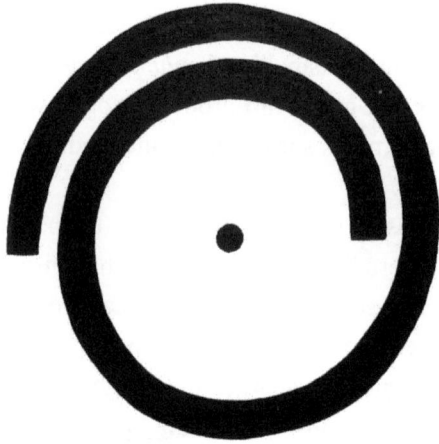

Western Red Cedar *(Thuja plicata)*

Keyword: constancy

Colour: blue

Chakras: 5, 6

Mantra: SO GUY G'HUU DRRRUH

Note sequence: *Eb *C *C F F D C Eb Eb *C

Colour Sequence: violet - yellow - magenta - gold - white

Western Red Cedar *(Thuja plicata)*

The western red cedar is not a true cedar but is related to cypress and juniper families. This species can be identified by its pineapple-like scent and by its single upright leader stem.

The primary influence of this tree is the perception of the underlying silence, stillness or peace behind every possible experience; that there is a constant flow of energy and a connection beneath all the changeability of life. This is particularly focused on the experience of the ever-flowing and changing of the emotions so that we do not become overwhelmed by strong emotions.

With this alteration of perspective it becomes possible to see every experience - no matter what its quality - as a means to achieve one's place in the flow of life. Beliefs and attitudes that are to do with one's self-image and the ability to express love can affect the energy of the Heart meridian. This tree energy calms and soothes agitation from these sources that may otherwise impair the functions of this meridian.

The same process occurs at the level of the brow chakra where western red cedar can help to heal damage that has distorted the mental processes and the subtle perceptions. At the crown chakra this process becomes the protection of one's basic energy patterns. The individual is able to act in accord with their own spiritual nature rather than being swayed by others. There is also an increased energy to allow change when it is necessary and to bring in dynamic activity to transform and grow.

This essence will help those whose relationships with others is unbalanced - either because they rely too much on the approval of others and who are continually drained emotionally by others, or, on the other hand, those people who do not register or ignore the feelings of others. There is an openness to other levels of knowledge and experience that increases energy to the whole system and frees the individual up to new ways of perceiving and acting. This has an overall effect on the subtle anatomy of the body, helping it to relax.

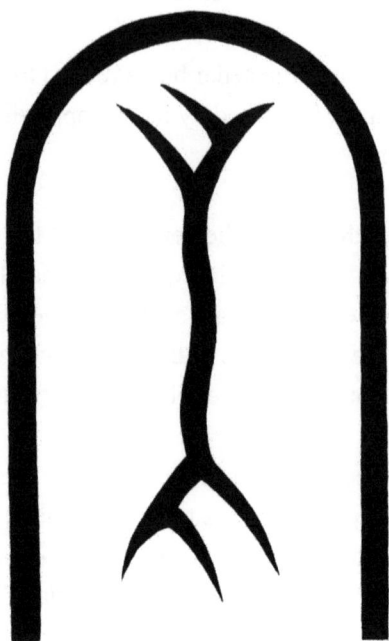

Whitebeam *(Sorbus aria)*

Keyword: Otherworlds

Colour: indigo

Chakras: 6, 7

Mantra: LAID TOO

Note sequence: C* C G F C* C G F

Colour sequence: red - violet- rich yellow

Whitebeam *(Sorbus aria)*

Whitebeam is native to limestone and chalk landscapes, though because of its modest, neat size, resistance to pollution and attractive appearance it is widely planted in town streets and parks. Whitebeam can grow to 80ft (24m) in these situations, though it is usually smaller in the wild.

It is an easily identified tree with large oval leaves that have green-grey hairy undersides. In early spring the light green buds appear like candle flames. When the new leaves are fully unfurled the umbels of creamy upright flowers open in May. These will ripen into bright scarlet berries that are rapidly eaten by birds.

Whitebeam stimulates fine levels of perception. It will energise the sacral, heart and brow chakras and a minor chakra just above the medulla oblongata, helping to balance creativity and insight with a keen awareness and alertness.

The mental and astral bodies are aligned to work with fine perceptions, so that one can begin to learn how to shift energy levels. Whitebeam brings a deeper attachment and understanding of the animal and plant kingdoms. It can also encourage contact and understanding of the natural world from the desire to be of service and to heal.

The essence increases one's harmony with cosmic energies and it opens the heart to recognise the underlying energy that supports all life. Whitebeam in this way strengthens the personal field whilst at the same time opening it up to experience, or float between other dimensions or angles of reality. A fine tuning of the energy fields occurs so as to be able to see and hear what is usually hidden.

The ephemeral shimmering of whitebeam's large soft leaves on a sunny spring day, where the large creamy flowers are showing, makes the tree appear otherworldly, as if it is not quite all within the physical reality.

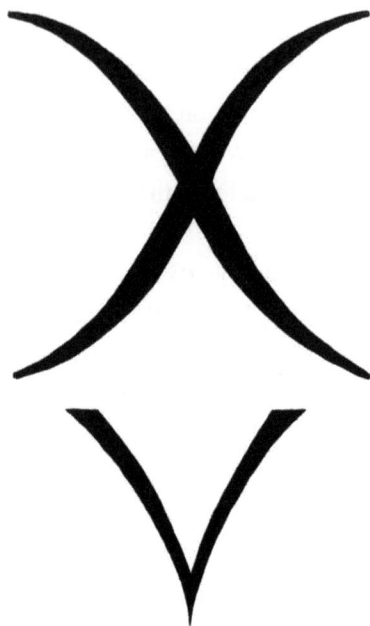

White Poplar *(Populus alba)*

Keywords: starting again

Colour: pink

Chakra: 4

Mantra: N'GAI B'HOO

Note sequence: C* B D D F C

Colour sequence: white - blue

White Poplar *(Populus alba)*

White poplar originates from the southern parts of Europe and western Asia. The date of its introduction to Britain is unknown but white poplar has certainly been planted as an ornamental tree since the 16th century. It rarely grows above 65ft (20m) and tends to have a leaning trunk and an asymmetrical crown. Like all poplars the leaves tremble in the breeze, and the almost white undersides create a silvery shimmering. The bark too, is easily identified: the upper trunk is silver with dark lozenge or nail-head markings. Both male and female flowers are woolly catkins. The males are crimson and the females are green and appear on separate trees before the leaves appear.

White poplar essence brings the security from which to grow outwards, express oneself and find new ways of being and thinking. Once there is established this sure foundation in confidence and self-worth it becomes easier to explore many different possibilities.

White poplar energises and heals the heart chakra so that there is an increased determination to recover from setbacks - particularly where they are of an emotional nature. Relationships, both with others and with oneself, are given a boost of energy through practical growth and expansiveness.

There is wisdom, intelligent energy, creativity and healing focused on how one sees the world and one's place in the world. White poplar can bring the ability to make positive changes that are new directions, perhaps not thought of before, and more in line with one's true desires and strengths.

Overall the essence brings an increase of wisdom, joy and contentment.

The alternation of dark green upper leaves and silver-white lower surfaces; the dark lower bark and the patterned upper trunk, both suggest a transformation of emotional states.

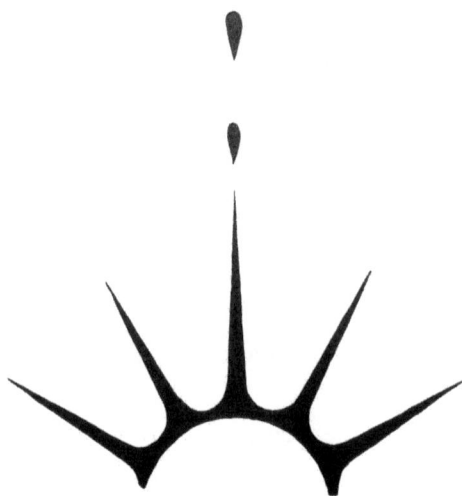

White Willow *(Salix alba)*

Keywords: true self

Colour: violet

Chakras: 3, 7

Mantra: TAANG UH TA' UNG UH

Note Sequence: D E D G B G D *B *E

Colour Sequence: gold - turquoise - red - infinitely fast vibration

White Willow *(Salix alba)*

White willow is the largest of the British willows growing to 80ft (25m) and forming an open, but often narrow crown of large boughs. The long thin leaves have silvery hairs that are particularly dense on the undersides giving the tree its characteristic colour.

White willow is characterised by the understanding and development of awareness of the whole being. It is able to access deep levels of knowledge, communication and devotion at many dimensional levels.

The solar plexus chakra is brought more energy that allows it to cleanse itself. This is at a level of a subtle cleansing, balancing the complementary energies of spirit and matter, energising the finest areas of potential and nudging them towards physical manifestation. In this particular combination, spirit is more enabled to infuse the individual being so that the influence of the smaller self, or ego, is taken out of the equation. When the personal influence lessens it is easier to become a clear channel for more universal energies.

The brow chakra is supported and its qualities enhanced. There is a greater clarification of all levels of communication and understanding, and the mental processes are allowed to perceive finer levels of reality. Smaller chakras at the medulla oblongata and centre of the forehead are also activated resulting in the ability to see oneself within a broader perspective, as part of a larger pattern. This allows the self to be brought to a truer balance. It also helps to prevent incorrect assumptions or arrogance about one's state of knowledge. White willow will balance those aspects of life that are either too narrowly fixed on a mundane level or too rarefied at a spiritual level. It will bring a more balanced vision of life in all its aspects.

Overall, there is a clarification and clearing of one's relationship to the universe, to the whole. With this can be experienced a sense of bliss or bliss consciousness, with love welling up to flavour all perceptions with its integrating energy.

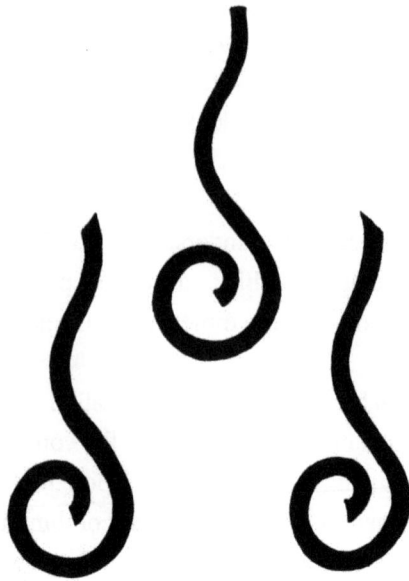

Wild Service Tree *(Sorbus torminalis)*

Keyword: unfolding

Colour: indigo

Chakra: 6

Mantra : AAA   CHAY

Note Sequence: G D G B

Colour Sequence: green - violet - yellow - blue - green

Wild Service Tree *(Sorbus torminalis)*

The wild service tree is a native of the British Isles but these days it is a rare sight, both because it favours ancient woodland and because it superficially resembles a small maple from a distance. The distribution of wild service tree is very localised in Britain, though more common on Continental Europe.

Wild service tree directs its energy to the expansion of awareness and the growth of clarity. There is a natural tendency to calm fears and restore the balance of mind. This naturally arises where there is a clearer picture about what is driving our behaviour - the reasons why we act or behave in the way we do.

This tree helps the Heart meridian to correct and balance for an effective deep healing of any long-standing emotional trauma. Such deep patterns or fractures of stress, unless released, set up permanent echoes which have a habit of repeating again and again. Thus, past life issues and past life emotional trauma can be greatly alleviated by this essence.

Equilibrium and calm also infuses the Gall Bladder meridian and this clarifies our needs and desires. Emotional stress at the sacral chakra is reduced. There is an increase in peacefulness, which allows personal creativity to emerge. There is also an increase in the ability to express oneself. Minor chakras at the ends of the fingers and toes help us to become more sensitive to the energies around us and allow access and use of healing energies. Wild service tree helps to activate these chakra points in a balanced way. Imbalances here may be indicated by a rejection of other people's energy or a tendency to unconsciously draw energy from others, leaving them feeling drained.

Wild service tree creates a degree of silence, like a blanket, over emotional noise. It does not prevent or sedate the flow of emotions or of thoughts, but it places the awareness in a state where these are no longer an obstruction to experiencing quietness.

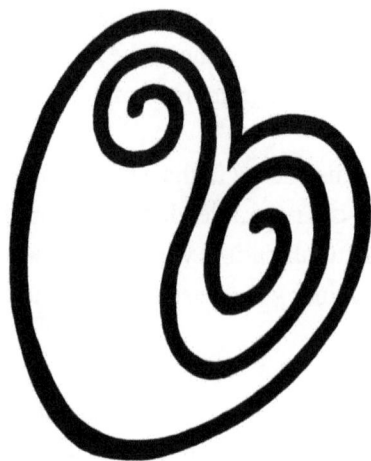

Willow Leaved Pear *(Pyrus salicifolia)*

Keywords: dance of life

Colours: red, orange

Chakra: 2

Mantra: AY TOO

Note Sequence: F# D Eb F#

Colour Sequence: cream white - blue - orange

Willow Leaved Pear *(Pyrus salicifolia)*

Willow-leaved pear is quite a common sight as a garden and park tree, particularly the weeping form *Pendula*. Willow-leaved pear is native to Siberia, Persia and the Caucasus where it grows on woodland margins and in thickets.

With the energy of willow-leaved pear comes a profound sense of security in oneself. This makes it possible to accept change without upset. There is an increased contentment, ease and experience of joy. Better self-awareness and flexibility give a greater possibility to act with wisdom, attuning to circumstances as they present themselves.

Willow-leaved pear focuses on clearing, detoxifying, healing and purifying. This makes it a useful essence during and after periods of illness. The Governing meridian is stimulated resulting in a more joyous expression of energy, greater dynamism, confidence and a sharper assessment of possible risks. It also helps to temper strong and inappropriate emotional reactions by reducing frustration and anger. The Circulation-Sex meridian (also known as Heart Protector or Pericardium meridian) is a focus whenever a new start is required, especially in an emotional relationship where greater self-confidence and self-awareness allows the change to be made wisely. Fears that arise from sexuality and relationship issues are lessened.

The solar plexus chakra, in particular, is energised by this tree enabling access to finer levels of perception and intuition that help to show up what is needed to achieve growth. It becomes much easier to communicate desires and wishes, ideas and instructions to others in order to achieve personal goals. Minor chakras are stimulated that increase self-worth and the ability to stand up for oneself. Willow-leaved pear brings the mind to a better state of clarity and open-mindedness, cleansed of all unwanted thoughts. There is the ability to see things clearly for what they are, with no illusions.
 At fine spiritual levels there is integration of life-energy. The dance of life is felt within and is able to be expressed to others. Enjoyment of existence is vital to our continued existence.

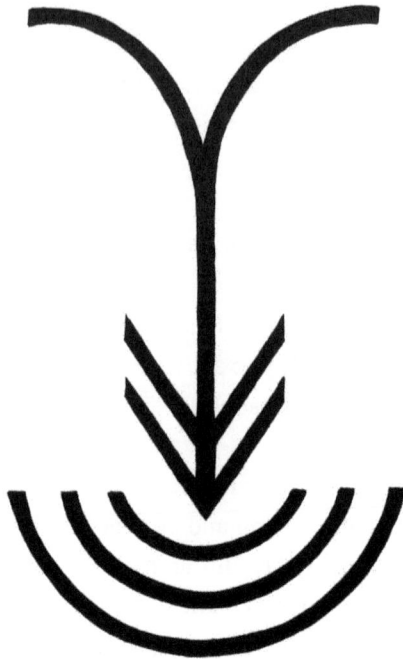

Wych Elm *(Ulmus glabra)*

Keyword: attainment

Colours: yellow, violet

Chakras: 3, 7

Mantra: PRRRUH GHAY TOE MOON GOO VO

Note Sequence: E C# F D G

Colour Sequence: indigo - white - pink - black - indigo

Wych Elm *(Ulmus glabra)*

The wych elm, also known as the mountain elm, is native to the British Isles and grows further north than any other elm. It thrives on deep, damp soils. The leaves are hairy and very rough to the touch, have a clearly pointed tip and a very unequal base. Wych elm, given the space, is a much wider tree than other elms but grows less tall with a maximum of about 100ft (30m). The flowers open on the shoots in February and March developing into apple-green bunches of seed cases, clearly visible before the leaves emerge. Wych elm is resistant to city pollution and so was widely planted in the towns of Scotland.

The essence of wych elm helps to bring the mind to clarity, allowing analysis and understanding of subtle thought processes. This makes it a useful energy to employ in any study situation. Organisation and expression of material becomes easier as the logical and intuitive parts of the mind work side by side.

There is a positive, more life-affirming outlook and a lifting of mood that would be helpful where there is pessimism or depression.

The Gallbladder meridian is strengthened in such a way that there can be a clear assessment of one's worth and place in the world. Wych elm brings a confidence in personal abilities and strengths.

Of the subtle bodies, the emotional body is most affected. There is a greater calm and balance within which it becomes very much easier to get thoughts and feelings across to others.

At a spiritual level, wych elm increases the ability to communicate and understand many different aspects of universal energy. There is a growth in peaceful awareness, no matter what state one is experiencing at the time. Wych elm can be used for meditation as it not only creates stable awareness but allows the consciousness to touch many subtle realms.

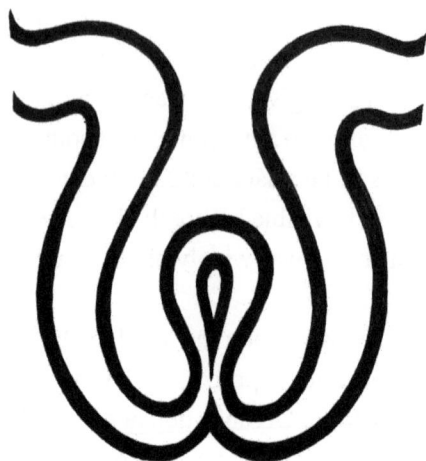

Yellow Buckeye *(Aesculus flava)*

Keyword: devas

Colour: indigo

Chakra: 7

Mantra: DUS HUH YIH RRNUH

Note Sequence: E C G D A

Colour Sequence: red - gold - blue - violet - deepest midnight blue

Yellow Buckeye *(Aesculus flava)*

Yellow buckeye, also called sweet buckeye, is superficially similar to horse chestnut though smaller in size. The crown narrows and the smooth trunk carries twisting, drooping branches with palmate leaves. In spring, the yellow flowers are produced in candle-like clusters.

The buckeyes are native to the river valleys of the eastern United States along the Ohio River and among the Allegheny and Appalachian Mountains. It was introduced into Britain in the mid 18th century.

There is an integration and harmony between the environment and one's interior energy systems. At the level of feeling there is a correspondence and interchange between oneself and one's surroundings. This forms easier links to devic energies and the ability to understand and integrate that level of consciousness.

The tree itself tends to act as a focus for anchoring devas to a location so it naturally augments contact with devic and elemental levels.

The crown chakra is enabled to understand different levels of communication and thought. There is the ability to frame new images and concepts in a logical, understandable way. The spiritual body is similarly tuned.

At the level of emotion, there is an activation of enthusiasm, drive and comprehending one's true needs.

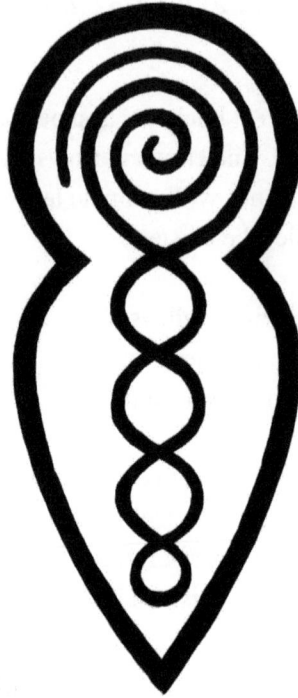

Yew *(Taxus baccata, Taxus baccata 'fastigiata')*

Keyword: protection

Colour: dark red

Chakras: Earth Star, 1

Mantra: DOW DAY VOW DAA

Note sequence: B Eb B C

Colour sequence: indigo - red - orange - yellow

Yew *(Taxus baccata, Taxus baccata 'fastigiata')*

The yew is among the most ancient of trees and is certainly the longest lived tree in Europe, if not the world. It is resistant to most pests and conditions except flood, and because of the inherent strength and flexibility of the wood, will carry large boughs without breaking. Yew is not a tall tree growing to about 50ft (15m), but where allowed it will spread widely resting its lower boughs on the ground and even re-rooting itself to send up daughter trees. A natural variety found by a farmer in County Fermanagh in the 1770's is the origin of the Irish yew, a stately towering upright yew with many straight 'spires' All Irish yews derive from this single find in the wild.

Yew essence is the paramount energy to use with all issues of survival and protection. Depending on the status of the individual system yew essence can either increase or regulate available energy levels. As it is profoundly grounding, those who are unused to being grounded may take some time to adjust to the differences of feeling and perception.

The root chakra is enlivened with all the resultant qualities that brings: increased motivation, drive, energy, practicality, strength and focus on the present, as well as protection from external energy intrusions. The solar plexus chakra also is enhanced, and together these chakras protect from harm by activating the highest spiritual values of survival and protection. This includes the activation of far memory, discrimination skills and deeper understanding of one's relationship to the planet and to the sun and its energy influence.

Once securely rooted into the planetary field it becomes possible with yew essence to explore many different times and places, accessing patterns held within the land and within the yew tree itself. This often directs the energy to the brow chakra where visionary experiences are processed and perceived.

The longevity and ability of yew trees to put on new growth, even after apparent death. The flexibility and strength of the wood and its red colouration.

Japanese Trees

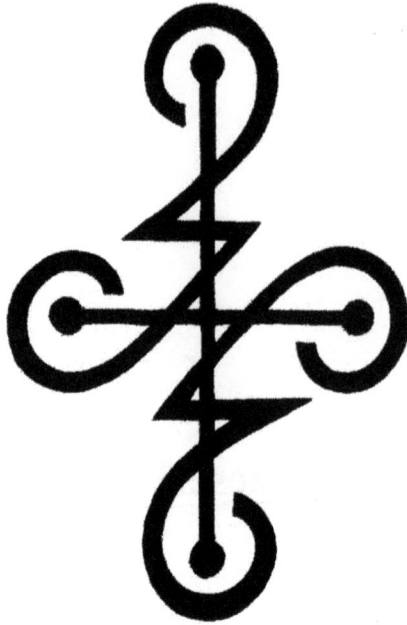

Buddhist Pine (Inumaki, Kusamaki) Big Leaf Podocarp.
Podocarpus macrophyllus,

Keywords: path of peace

Colour: violet

Chakra: 7

Mantra: SHAU SHAU SHAU

Note Sequence: G *D *F# *D

Colour Sequence: indigo - yellow - white - yellow - violet

Buddhist Pine (Inumaki, Kusamaki) Big Leaf Podocarp.
(Podocarpus macrophyllus)

The Japanese name, Kusamaki, is being increasingly used as a replacement for Buddhist Pine, a common name that is not accurate as the tree is not a member of the Pine Family.

A small or medium-sized evergreen tree up to 20m. The leaves are deep green, 6-12cm long and 1cm broad with a central rib. It has cone that matures into fleshy, reddish purple berries. The flesh of these is edible, though the inner seeds are not. It grows in forests, thickets and roadsides up to 1000m.

Kusamaki is the State tree of Chiba Prefecture. It is preferred for house building in Okinawa because of its resistance to termites and water damage. It is very important to Chinese feng shui. Its Chinese and English names derive from its frequent planting within shrines and temple grounds.

 Useful when there is anxiety that prevents action; when there is fear of death; where there is avoidance of contact and interaction in the world.

A release of fears and an ability to enjoy the experiences of life.

Increased sense of safety and confidence in one's abilities.

Ability to carry out actions in an organised and wise manner.

Communication is truthful and clear, encouraging peace and a broad perspective.

Clarity in personal path and personal expression.

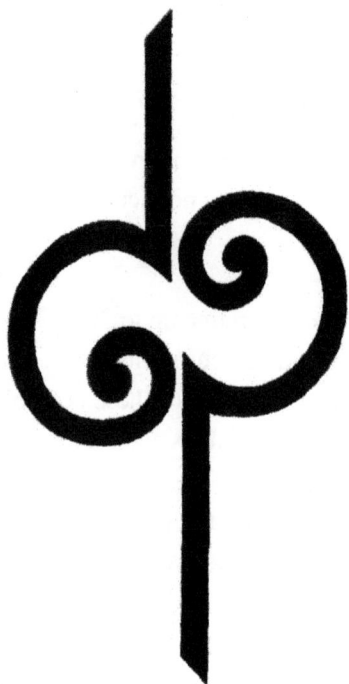

Candleberry Tree (Nanzin Haze)
Chinese tallow tree, Florida aspen, chicken tree, grey popcorn tree,
candleberry tree. *(Sapium sebiferum)*

Keyword: emergence

Colour: white

Chakras: 2, 7

Mantra: BUH HOH PUH HEE

Note Sequence: C# *F# F# G

Colour Sequence: indigo - blue - violet - white - red.

Candleberry Tree (Nanzin Haze)

Chinese tallow tree, Florida aspen, chicken tree, grey popcorn tree, candleberry tree. *(Sapium sebiferum)*

These latter names reflect its introduction and spread in the south-east of the USA where it is regarded as somewhat a nuisance because of its fast-growing profusion. It is classed as 'noxious'. Sap and leaves are said to be toxic, but the tree also has very useful properties - its seeds are coated in a waxy substance used for candle-making and for soap.

It is the third most productive source of bio-diesel in the world. The nectar makes high quality, copious honey. The tree, native to eastern Asia, grows throughout Japan in all conditions except deep shade.

It has elegant leaves resembling the bo tree *(Ficus religiosa)*, bright green above, paler below. The tree produces long spikes of yellow-green and white flowers that ripen into three-lobed capsules. In autumn the leaves can become bright yellow, orange, purple and red.

 A sense of unfolding and renewing.
The clearing away of anything unnecessary.
Energy to begin again. Protection during delicate times of growth.
Making space for new starts.
Confidence to rest in silence.
Gentle healing and purifying.

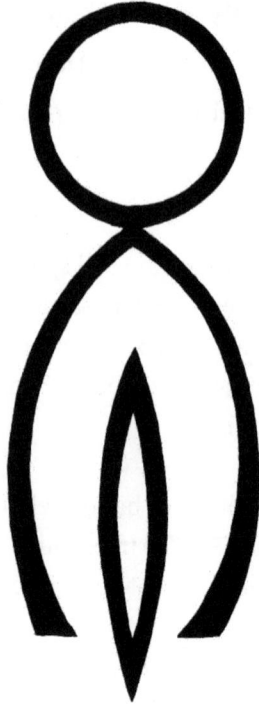

Camellia (Yabutsubaki)
Japanese camellia, rose of winter *(Camellia japonicum)*

Keywords: settled down

Colour: pink

Chakras: 2, 4

Mantra: ROO CHI HAA ROO

Note Sequence: F# *Eb E *Eb

Colour Sequence: violet - red - magenta - white

Camellia (Yabutsubaki)
Japanese camellia, rose of winter. *(Camellia japonicum)*

A small tree or flowering shrub up to 6m (20ft), native to southern areas of Japan, Korea and China. It is a forest tree growing between 1,000 and 3,000 ft. In the wild camellia flowers between January and March bearing pink or white flowers with six or seven petals clustered close to each branch. The fruit is a round capsule with three compartments, each containing one or two large brown seeds. Cultivated varieties have many more flower petals.

Freedom from the pressures of others, freedom from troubles.
 Peaceful and easy relationship to self and others.
Using past experiences to solve problems.
Relaxing of rigid ideas. Increased tolerance and patience.
Quiet individuality.
Seeing the best in everything

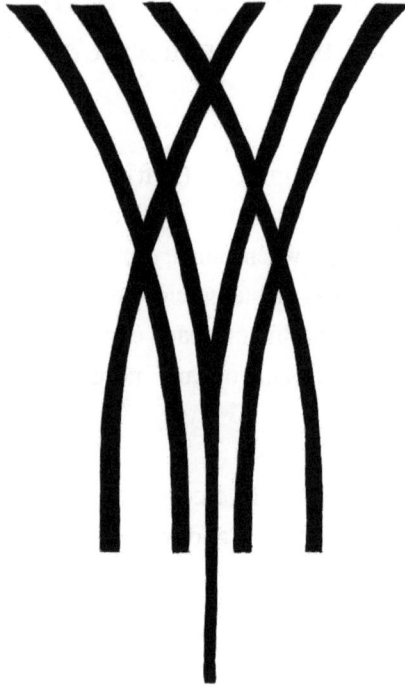

Camphor Tree (Kusunoki)
camphor wood, camphor laurel, Ho wood. *(Cinnamomum camphora)*

Keyword: idea

Colour: orange

Chakra: 2

Mantra: SHAA KOO TUH HAY TUH HAY TAH

Note Sequence: Ab *G G *E

Colour Sequence: gold - violet - indigo - gold.

Camphor Tree (Kusunoki)
camphor wood, camphor laurel, Ho wood *(Cinnamomum camphora)*

This is native to China, Japan and Taiwan. It is a large, evergreen tree
(20-30m). It has rough, vertically fissured pale bark. In some ways it
resembles the sturdiness and solidity of the oak. Leaves are glossy and waxy,
smelling of camphor when crushed. In spring there is a profusion of clusters of
small white flowers that ripen into black, berry-like fruit.

All parts of the camphor tree contain volatile essential oils, which are extracted
by steam distillation from leaves and wood. Trees in different areas contain
unique chemical signatures. Japanese trees tend to be high in linalools, in India
camphor is dominant, in Madagascar 1-8 cineole is extracted as ravintsara.
This oil (often confused with ravensara), is better for children than the more
powerful ravensera (*Ravensera anisata* - which has a higher camphor content).

Camphor wood can be chipped and steamed to crystallise the white substance
in a solid, waxy form. It has been used in cooking, incense and medicine. It
also acts as an insect repellent and flea-killer.

Becoming aware of the inherent intelligence of the body.
Knowing what is useful and what needs to be avoided.
Making the best choices, enabling one to succeed.
Healing deep hurts allowing renewal.
Bringing about the best circumstances for creativity and healing.

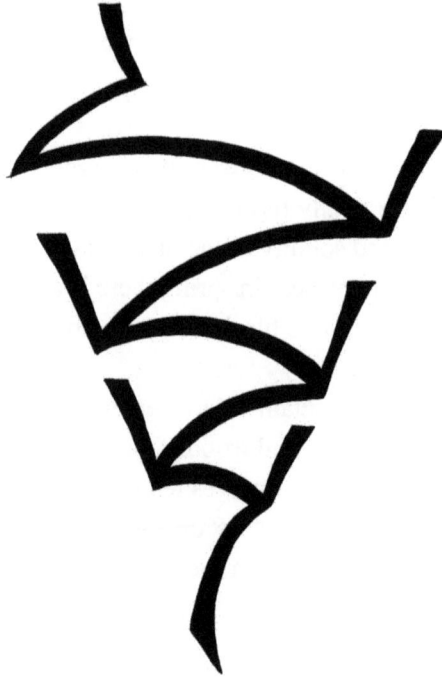

Kuosa dogwood (Yamaboushi) *(Cornus kuosa)*

Keyword: holding

Colour: red

Chakra: 1

Mantra: SHOO G'HOO J'HEE. T'HOW RROO

Note Sequence: G   G   G   *Eb   F

Colour Sequence: turquoise - blue - dark blue - blue

Kuosa dogwood (Yamaboushi)
(Cornus kuosa)

Cornus kuosa, also called Kuosa dogwood, Chinese dogwood, Korean dogwood, Japanese dogwood. It is a small, deciduous tree up to 12m tall, native to eastern Asia. It is easily distinguished from the flowering dogwood (*Cornus florida*), by a later flowering period and more pointed 'flower' petals. The bright, four-petalled, white flowers are, in fact, the bracts that surround the very small yellow-green flowers clustered in the centre. The fruit is a pink or red compound berry that can grow to 4cm. The fruit is very edible and is sometimes used in wine making.

Like most other dogwoods, Kuosa dogwood has simple, opposite leaves with prominent unbranched veins.

Anchored and grounded to access a personal source of energy.

Actions become integrated and powerful, calm and imaginative.

Strengthening of life-energy and a smooth flow of information between levels of Being.

Willing to be quiet and listen to fine levels of awareness.

Happy knowing that not everything can be known or understood.

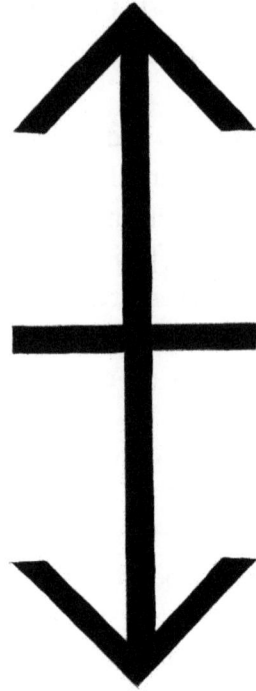

Hackberry (Enoki)
hackberry, nettle tree. *(Celtis sinensis)*

Keyword: evolution

Colour: violet

Chakra: 7

Mantra: FOE T'HUL UH RAY FOE T'HUL UH RAY

Note Sequence: D G A *D E

Colour Sequence: turquoise - violet - magenta - yellow - white.

Hackberry (Enoki)
hackberry, nettle tree. *(Celtis sinensis)*

This belongs to a genus of 60-70 hackberries that live in warm, temperate regions of the Northern Hemisphere. It is an ancient tree with fossil records from the Miocene Period in Europe.

The tree is medium-sized (10-25m) but often spreading. The trunk is smooth, grey and buttressed, somewhat resembling European beech. Leaves are rough, toothed and resemble the herb, nettle. Small flowers appear in early spring as the leaves develop. The fruit is a small drupe of round, sweet berries.

Accessing invisible worlds of spirit through the realms of nature.
Making sense of very subtle perceptions and levels of communication,
intuition, inspiration in practical ways in life.
Energy to expand; practical power; the drive to grow;
Using the dynamic force of Nature to find wholeness.
Space to grow and evolve.

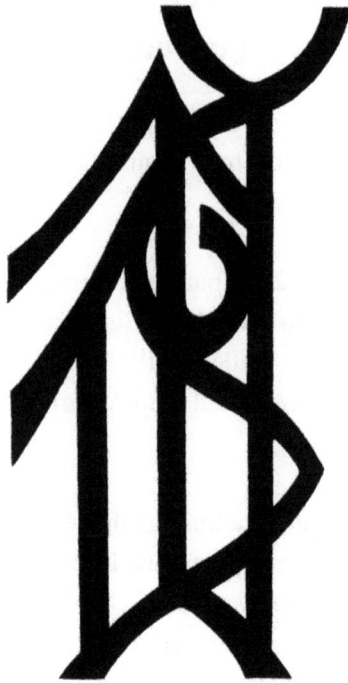

Hiba (Asuhi, Asunaro)
false arborvitae, hiba arborvitae *(Thujopsis dolobrata)*

Keyword: calm

Colour: blue

Chakras: 5, 6

Mantra: B'HOO AA VAA

Note Sequence: F Ab *D F

Colour Sequence: green - gold - blue - red.

Hiba (Asuhi, Asunaro)
false arborvitae, hiba arborvitae *(Thujopsis dolobrata)*

The common Japanese name, asunaro refers to the phrase: " Tomorrow it will become a hinoki", because its form resembles a young hinoki cypress, with a densely foliated conical shape.

It is a medium to large evergreen tree of the cypress Family (up to 40m) with a characteristic red-brown bark that peels in vertical strips. The leaves are fleshy and glossy green with white bands below. Its scent is similar to pineapple. Woody cones appear at the end of branches.

Hiba is drought-sensitive and loves high rainfall and moist soils. The wood, which is durable and scented is valuable, making it one of the Five Sacred Trees of Kiso.

Calming fears and anxieties.
Correct balance of mind.
Alert and receptive to subtle levels of communication.
Balanced state of personal energy.
Intuitive insight.
Accepting peace.
Quiet awareness, alert stillness.
Effective communication.

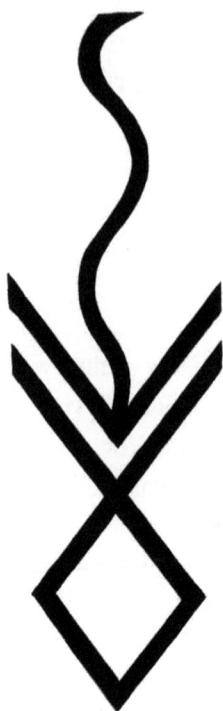

Hinoki (hinoki)
Japanese cypress. *(Chamaecyparis obtusa)*

Keyword: satisfaction

Colour: yellow

Chakra: 3

Mantra: UH T'HEE GUH

Note Sequence: D *C *A

Colour Sequence: violet - orange - gold - green

Hinoki
Japanese cypress *(Chamaecyparis obtusa)*

Hinoki cypress is one of the Five Sacred Trees of Kiso. Its timber has a rich, straight grain, light pinky-brown and is lemon-scented. It is very resistant to rot and is used extensively in palaces, temples and shrines, notably at Ise.

Like many cypresses, it has many cultivars that are used in ornamental gardens worldwide. The main differences between hinoki and sawara *(Chamaecyparis pisifera)*, is that hinoki has long, blunt-tipped scale-like leaves, whilst sawara has pointed leaf-tips.

Hinoki flowers are small buds at branch-tips with female flowers at the terminal tip. Hinoki is a slow-growing tree up to 35m preferring moist soils and cool summers. The bark is dark red-brown.

The ability to act in ways that bring increased happiness and contentment, and achievement of personal goals.
An increased calm and peace reducing agitation or lack of focus.
Channelling powerful drives and emotions.
Enlivening the senses, becoming alert and enthusiastic.
Integration of personal with universal life-energy.

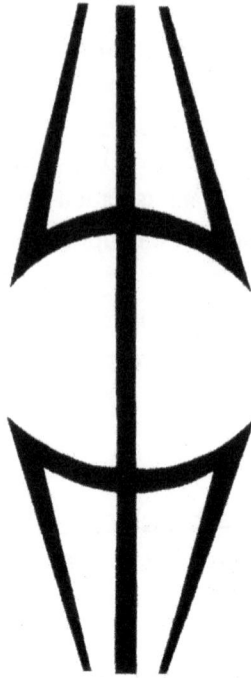

Holly Olive (Hi-ragi)
holly osmanthus, false holly, hihiragi. *(Osmanthus heterophyllus)*

Keywords: tranquil view

Colour: blue

Chakras: 5, 6

Mantra: D'HOO D'HO.

Note Sequence: E G A

Colour Sequence: indigo - blue - gold - pink

Holly Olive (Hi-ragi)
holly osmanthus, false holly, hihiragi *(Osmanthus heterophyllus)*

This is native to central and southern Japan. An evergreen shrub or small tree (up to 8m). Leaves are opposite and take two forms: upper leaves are smooth, glossy and entire, whilst lower leaves bear between one to four long, spine - tipped teeth on each side. The flowers are very fragrant, white and appear in the autumn. The fruit is an ovoid, dark purple drupe that ripens the following year.

In the Kojiki it is mentioned in relationship to Hihiragi-no-sono-hana-madzumi-no-kami ('Spirit waiting to see the flowers of the osmanthus'), and as a spear of osmanthus wood given from the Emperor to Prince Yamatotake before he leaves to subdue the east.

Peace that allows deep insight.
Seeing ways beyond states of unhappiness.
Transformation of anger and other strong, imbalanced emotions.
Security within oneself.
Inspiration and flow of life-energy.
Activation of personal potential, protection of core energies.
Reduction of all frictions.

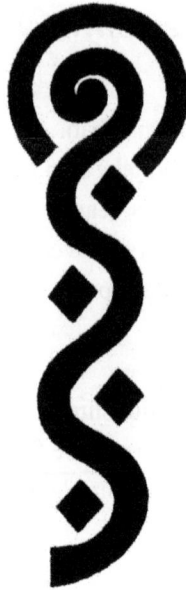

Japanese Cherry (Sakura)
(Prunus serrulata)

Keyword: unity

Colour: pink

Chakra: 4

Mantra: DHAU TIH DAA VAA DUU

Note Sequence: C A G

Colour Sequence: indigo - orange - red - magenta - white - magenta - ultraviolet.

Japanese Cherry (Sakura)
(Prunus serrulata)

The Japanese cherry, sakura has well over 200 cultivars in Japan. Cherry blossom has long been a potent symbol here - both as a national emblem and as a symbol of the ephemeral beauty of the world. The souls of the dead are sometimes equated with cherry blossom, particularly of warriors.

Cherries begin to blossom first in Okinawa in January, reaching Kyoto and Tokyo about the end of March or beginning of April.

Amongst the many varieties is *Prunus "Tai-Haku"*, an ancient Japanese cherry that had become extinct in Japan, reintroduced by a single tree found in a garden in Sussex, England. This variety has single white flowers. Known as the Great White Cherry, it grows to 12m (40ft).

Compassion and clarity, maintaining appropriate energy connections.
Relaxation and acceptance.
Openness and intuitive insight.
Calming fears, release of long-held stresses and blocks.
Supporting creativity and healing.
Peace and belonging.

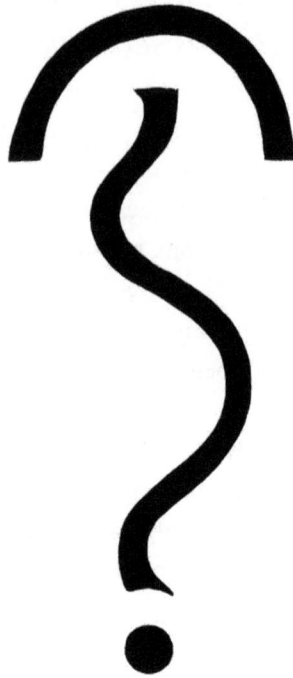

Japanese Hornbeam (Kumashide)
(Carpinus japonica)

Keyword: searching

Colour: orange

Chakras: 2, 4

Mantra: MAA GOW

Note Sequence: B   C   *D   *C   C

Colour Sequence: blue - pink - blue

Japanese Hornbeam (Kumashide)
"Carpinus japonica"

This is a variety of hornbeam native to Japan. It grows to 12 - 15m. And carries long, toothed leaves, each of which has 20-24 sunken veins. Every third tooth is whiskered. The leaves turn bright yellow in autumn. Tightly branched and spreading, it bears catkin-like flowers in spring before the leaves, which become small pendulous winged fruit, first green then brown.

Exploration of the personal path to power. Healing our relationship with the world and others. Restoring balance to the heart, relaxing the mind, calming anxieties and fears.
All energy systems become more efficient and organised, reducing stress levels. Clarity of personal direction.

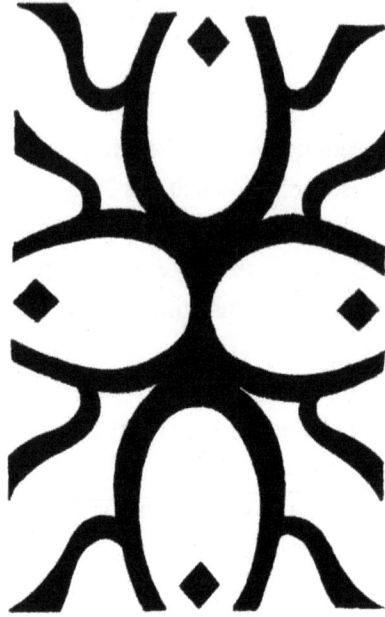

Japanese Maple (Yamamomiji, irohamomji, momiji)
(Acer palmatum)

Keyword: soothing

Colour: yellow

Chakras: 2, 3

Mantra: T'HAI

Note Sequence: B D *A B D

Colour Sequence: red - white - green - gold.

Japanese Maple (Yamamomiji, irohamomji, momiji)
(Acer palmatum)

This smooth Japanese maple, is a small tree reaching to 10m, occasionally to 16m. It is commonly found as an under-storey tree in woodland. Often many-stemmed it has a dome-like habit. Leaves are palmate with five, seven or nine deeply-cut pointed lobes. Flowers are small, opening in April in small clusters that turn into winged fruits (samara). Japanese maple shows great genetic variation. Seedlings from the same tree will often show differences of leaf size, shape and colour. This has been taken advantage of, and a great many cultivars have been developed. Branches and leaves are used in Traditional Chinese Medicine.

Healing, calming, soothing fears.
A flow of relaxation and understanding.
Creativity, playfulness and enjoyment.
Deep connections to the power of Nature.
Issues resolved to do with power, conflict and control.
Soothing flow of internal and external energies.

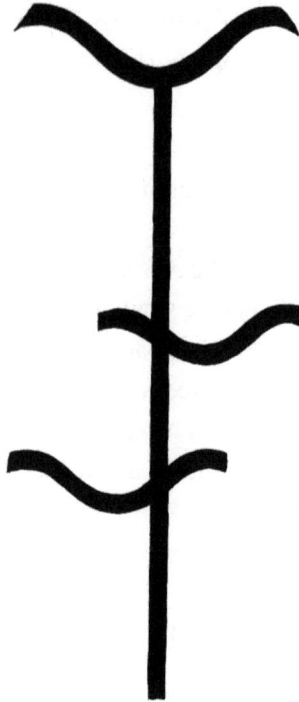

Japanese Cedar (Sugi)
(Cryptomera japonica)

Keywords: holding still, supporting all

Colour: orange

Chakra: 2

Mantra: D'HII POH G'HAA PIH

Note Sequence: G *C G

Colour Sequence: deep orange - blue - violet.

Japanese Cedar (Sugi)
(Cryptomera japonica)

Sugi is a conifer of the Cypress Family. There is only one species, and it is native exclusively to Japan. It is the national tree of Japan and takes pride of place around shrines and temples, where many magnificent ancient examples can be found.

Cryptomeria grows quickly in forests on deep, well-drained soils that have warm, moist conditions. It is intolerant of poor soils and cold, drier climates. It is a very large evergreen tree, reaching up to 70m (230 ft) tall with a 4m (13 ft) trunk diameter, with red-brown bark which peels in vertical strips. The leaves are arranged spirally and are curved and needle-like. The globular seed cones are found at the end of branchlets. Flowering is heavy in early spring (sugi and hinoki are the two greatest causes of hay-fever in Japan), turning the foliage a rusty red with pollen.

The discovery of balanced power.
Inner poise and calm.
Tolerance, relaxation, acceptance.
Support for positive actions, mediating between different viewpoints.
Creative space, creative silence, balanced awareness.

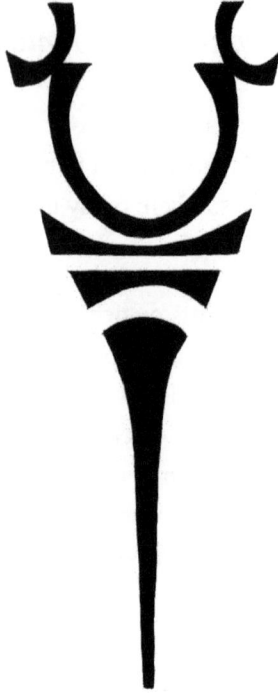

Katsura (Katsura)
Japanese katsura, Japanese judas tree.
(Cercidiphyllum japonicum)

Keyword: interpretation

Colour: blue

Chakras: 5, 6

Mantra: MAA LAA YUU JURRUH SAA

Note Sequence: A A *G *D F

Colour Sequence: blue -white - blue

Katsura (Katsura)
Japanese katsura, Japanese judas tree.
(Cercidiphyllum japonicum)

Katsura is the largest deciduous tree in China and Japan. It is a very ancient species with many primitive features. Trees are either male or female. Small, red male flowers are in tight bunches, female trees carry claw-like, dark red flowers that ripen into small pods.

There are two species of katsura, both native to Japan and China, *C. japanicum* and *C. magnificum,* of which the former has the larger range of habitat. Japanese katsura is a multi-stemmed tree growing to 40 - 50 metres. The bark is rough and furrowed. The leaves are heart-shaped on shorter branches, packed close together opposite each other. On longer branches the leaves are more elliptical and slightly toothed. Leaves tend to cover all branches right back to the trunk. Katsura has impressive autumn colours: rich reds, yellows, pinks and oranges all with a strong, sugary scent. It is a fast-growing tree but needs deep, wet soil. In dry conditions it can lose all its leaves and will put out new foliage when conditions improve.

C. magnificum is found in central Honshu where it grows at higher altitudes than *C. japonicum.* It is a smaller tree, growing up to 10m, with smooth bark and longer leaves.

Brings a clearer view of every situation, the possible developments and significance.
Actions that are appropriate and sufficiently detached from personal emotions and concerns.
Intuitive and imaginative skills used to bring healing and understanding.
Caring for others without taking on their suffering.
Acceptance of change because one is grounded and protected.

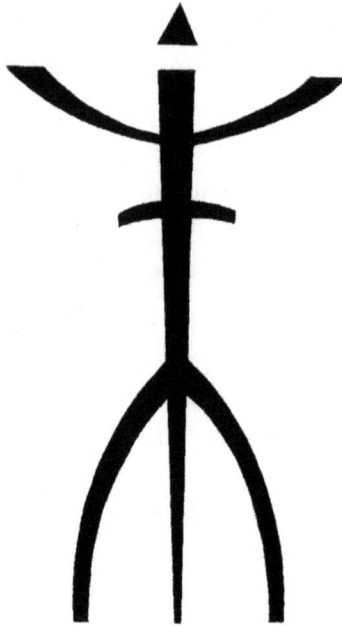

Keaki (Keyaki)
Japanese Zelkova, keyaki; ju shu,
(Zelkova serrata)

Keyword: friendship

Colour: green

Chakra: 4

Mantra: PLUH VAH D'HAA INGOH

Note Sequence: C *A *G C

Colour Sequence: gold - pink - indigo - blue-green - yellow.

Keaki   (Keyaki)
Japanese Zelkova, keyaki; ju shu,
(Zelkova serrata)

This is a species of zelkova native to Japan, Korea, eastern China, and Taiwan. It is often grown as an ornamental tree, and is used in bonsai.

It is a medium sized deciduous tree usually growing to 30 m. (100 ft). It has a short trunk dividing into many upright and erect spreading stems forming a broad, round topped head. The tree grows rapidly when young though the growth rate slows as it matures.

 The leaves are alternate, simple and ovate to oblong-ovate with toothed margins, to which the tree owes its species name, s*errata*.The leaves are rough on top and hairless on the underside. They are green to dark green in spring and throughout the summer, in autumn turning to shades of yellow, orange and red.

Keaki develops flowers in spring with the leaves.They are yellow-green, not showy, and occur in tight groups along new stems. They give rise to small, ovate, drupes that ripen in late summer to autumn from green to brown. Its twigs are slender with small, dark conical buds in a zigzag pattern. The bark is grayish white to grayish brown and either smooth with lenticels or exfoliating in patches to reveal orange inner bark. Branchlets are brownish purple to brown. Keaki prefers full to partial sun and prefers moist, well drained soils. Keaki trained with a single, central trunk are found often as street trees in Tokyo. Here the spreading upper branches make an elegant archway over the traffic.

Balancing the heart, improved relationship.
Increase in happiness.
Enjoyment of one's surroundings.
Improved self-image.
Clarity of mind and calmness of emotions.
Seeing what is true and valuable.
Letting go of illusion and misconceptions.

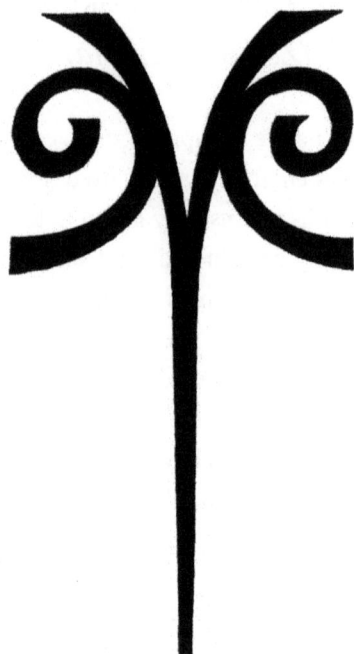

Myrtle-leaved Oak (Shirakashi)
shirakashi oak, bamboo leaf oak, Chinese evergreen oak
(Quercus myrsinifolia)

Keyword: dominion

Colour: gold

Chakras: 3, 4

Mantra: NAA JAYI KII BRRRUH

Note Sequence: Eb F# F# C

Colour Sequence: blue - gold - white - green - red.

Myrtle-leaved Oak (Shirakashi)
shirakashi oak, bamboo leaf oak, Chinese evergreen oak
(Quercus myrsinifolia)

Shirakashi oak, is an evergreen oak tree growing to 20 metres (66 ft) tall. It is native to east central and southeast China, Japan, Korea, Laos, Northern Thailand, and Vietnam.

Quercus myrsinifolia is a small, domed, evergreen tree, occasionally multi stemmed. Its leathery, hairless leaves are narrow, lanceolate, up to 12cm long, dark green above and slightly glaucous beneath. The newly emerged leaves have a purple/ bronze colour. The bark is dark, pinkish grey, smooth, occasionally with thin orange furrows. The flowers are pistillate flowers on young shoots, with 2 to 6 being borne on a slender stem. The fruit is an acorn, being borne in clusters of 2 to 6 on a long stem. This tree is not grazed by rabbits or deer.

Protection from outside disruption.
Appropriate levels of energy and information.
Relaxed strength.
Good results and success in action.
Understanding the flow of manifestation.
Supporting individual goals.
Vigilance, self- reliance, mastery.

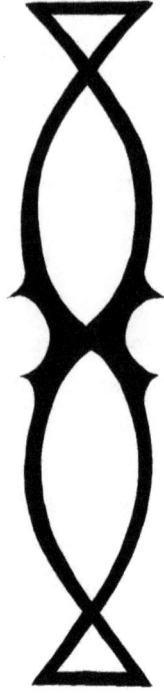

Pagoda Tree (enju, esozugu)
scholar tree, huai
(Sophora japonica)

Keyword: determination

Colour: red

Chakra: 1

Mantra: THURUH KAI AA A

Note Sequence: G   A   Bb

Colour Sequence: light green - white - pink - violet.

Pagoda Tree (enju, esozugu)
scholar tree, huai
(Sophora japonica)

Japanese pagoda tree was introduced into Japan from China. It got the name 'scholar tree' because a schoolmaster was of sufficient rank to have this tree planted on his grave. This tree belongs to the Family *Leguminosae* and resembles the Black locust tree (*Robinia spp.*). It grows to 25m. It has warm brown bark and bright blue-green shoots. Leaves are pointed leaflets arranges in pairs with a terminal single leaflet, bright green with downy undersides. Creamy white, fragrant flowers, resembling those of the pea, appear in late summer hanging in long panicles, ripening into long pods.

All parts of the tree are important in Traditional Chinese Medicine. It is an anti-bacteriological bitter for improved blood and liver functions and removal of intestinal parasites.

Cleverness and skill used in original ways.
Knowing how one can live and prosper.
Eloquent, wise communication.
Ability to face the unknown with peace and acceptance.
New ideas, new abilities to organise and structure one's surroundings.

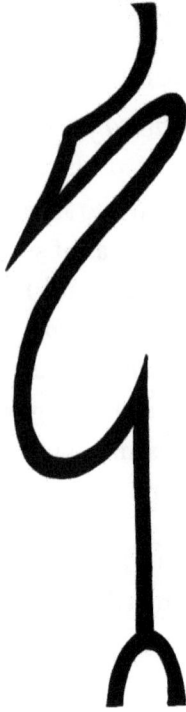

Pieris (asebi)
Japanese andromeda, lily of the valley shrub,
(Pieris japonica)

Keyword: humility

Colour: orange

Chakra: 2

Mantra: DAY NAA TEE

Note Sequence: G C *D E

Colour Sequence: violet.

Pieris (asebi)
Japanese andromeda, lily of the valley shrub,
(Pieris japonica)

It is native to eastern China, Taiwan, and Japan where it grows in mountain thickets. *Pieris japonica* is a shrub or a small tree, a member of the Heath Family *(Ericaceae)*. It grows to 1–4 m. tall, occasionally up to 10m. with alternate, simple leaves on brittle stems. The fragrant, bell-shaped flowers are white and borne in early spring in long clusters. Flower buds are pink, new foliage is coppery-red turning to glossy green. The bark is red-brown becoming split and scaly with age. Pieris has been widely cultivated for gardens as it provides colour and interest throughout the year.

All parts of the plant are very poisonous, with small amounts likely to be lethal. Leaves and flower nectar, (including honey), contain the toxins that can cause heart failure, paralysis and convulsions.

Personal growth and abundance achieved through flexibility and taking advantage of what is present.
Acceptance of obligations and abilities.
Trust and quiet confidence in oneself.
Satisfaction and fulfilment within the constraints of one's life.
Protection from stresses.

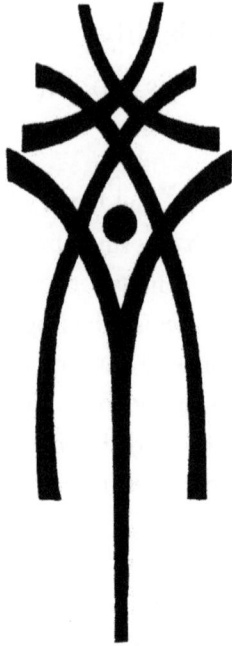

Sakaki
shrine offering tree
(Cleyera japonica)

Keyword: offering

Colours: red, indigo

Chakras: 1, 6

Mantra: DAY NEH KO VOW

Note Sequence: A F G A A

Colour Sequence: gold - red - white.

Sakaki
shrine offering tree
(Cleyera japonica)

Sakaki is a flowering evergreen tree native to warm areas of Japan, Korea and mainland China. It can reach a height of 10 m. The leaves are 6–10 cm long, smooth, oval, leathery, shiny and dark green above, yellowish-green below, with deep furrows for the leaf stem. The bark is dark reddish brown and smooth. The small, scented, cream-white flowers open in early summer, and are followed later by berries which start red and turn black when ripe. Sakaki is one of the common trees in the second layer of the evergreen oak forests. Sakaki is a most important tree in Shinto, linked to the enticing of Amaterasu from her cave and used extensively both in offerings to the spirits, *kami,* and as demarcation of sacred spaces and boundaries.

 Sakaki wood is used for making utensils (especially combs), building materials, and fuel. It is commonly planted in gardens, parks, and shrines.

Considered, balanced action.

Harmonious power.

Insight, judgement, understanding.

Actions that bring harmony.

Increasing quiet and peace of mind.

Ability to receive and understand communication from the deep levels of the mind.

Meditative silence.

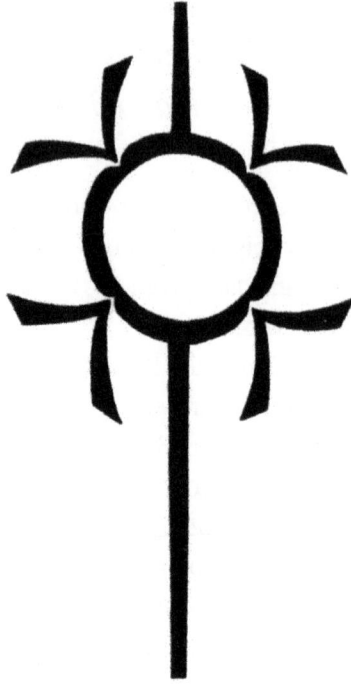

Sweet Osmanthus (Kinmokusei)
sweet olive, tea olive, fragrant olive.
(Osmanthus fragrans)

Keyword: expression

Colour: indigo

Chakra: 6

Mantra: OWE NYIH T'HAA TEH

Note Sequence: F# A A B

Colour Sequence: pink - gold - orange - indigo - yellow.

Sweet Osmanthus (Kinmokusei)
sweet olive, tea olive, fragrant olive.
(Osmanthus fragrans)

This is a species of osmanthus native to Asia, from the Himalayas east through southern China, Taiwan to southern Japan. It is an evergreen shrub or small tree growing 3-12 m tall. The leaves are 7-15 cm long and 2.6-5 cm broad, with an entire or finely toothed margin. The small flowers are white, pale yellow, yellow, or orange-yellow, small (1 cm long), with a strong fragrance and they are produced in small clusters in the late summer and autumn. The fruit is a purple-black drupe 10-15 mm long containing a single hard-shelled seed; it is mature in the spring about six months after flowering.

Sweet osmanthus is cultivated as an ornamental plant in gardens for its deliciously fragrant flowers which carry the scent of ripe peaches or apricots. A number of cultivars, with different flower colours are available for gardens. In China the flowers are added to tea to create *gui hua* cha scented tea. They are also used to make osmanthus scented jam, sweet cakes, dumplings, soups and alcoholic drinks. In North India the flowers are used to protect clothes from insect damage.

Considerate and elegant communication.
Creative, meditative states.
Experiencing peace and being able to communicate this effectively.
Flowing along one's true path.
Release of trauma and past-life stresses.

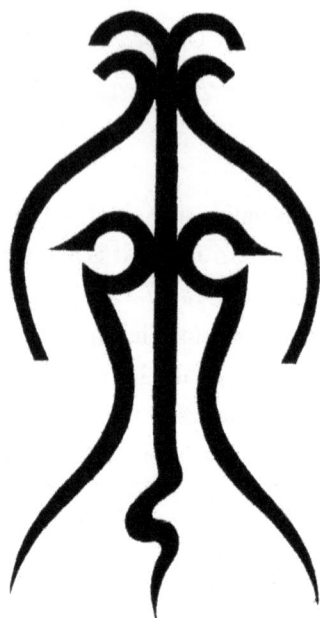

Wisteria (Fuji)
(also spelled Wistaria or Wysteria)
(Wisteria japonica)

Keyword: poise

Colour: indigo, violet

Chakras: 6, 7

Mantra: DOW TOE FAA

Note Sequence: A C# Eb G A

Colour Sequence: indigo - violet.

Wisteria (Fuji)
(also spelled Wistaria or Wysteria)
(Wisteria japonica)

This is a genus of flowering plants in the pea family, *Fabaceae,* that includes ten species of woody climbing vines native to the Eastern United States and to China, Korea, and Japan. Some species are popular ornamental plants, especially in China and Japan.

Wisteria vines climb by twining their stems either clockwise or counter-clockwise round any available support. They can climb as high as 20 m above the ground and spread out 10 m laterally. The world's largest known wisteria vine is in Sierra Madre, California. A Chinese wisteria planted in 1894, it covers more than 1 acre (0.40 ha). The largest wisteria in Japan is in Ashikaga Flower Park, Tochigi. Planted around 1870, in 2008 it covered approximately 1,990 square meters (0.5 acre).

The leaves of wisteria are alternate, 15 to 35 cm long and pointed with 9 to 19 leaflets. The flowers are produced in large racemes 10 to 80 cm long, similar to those of the genus Laburnum, but are purple, violet, pink or white. Flowering is in the spring (just before or as the leaves open) in some Asian species, and in mid to late summer in the American species and *W. japonica*. The flowers of some species are fragrant, especially Chinese Wisteria. The seeds are produced in pods similar to those of Laburnum, and, like the seeds of that genus, are poisonous.

Wisteria, especially *Wisteria sinensis*, is very hardy and fast-growing. They thrive in full sun. Wisteria has nitrogen fixing capability provided by *Rhizobia* bacteria in root nodules so can grow on poor soils.

Finding peace and harmony.
Creative action, elegance, charisma, poise.
Understanding power, confidence, perfect and appropriate expression.
Following personal path with integrity and peace.

APPENDICES

The Chakras

Over the last three thousand years sages, philosophers and mystics have
described the subtle energies in our environment and within our bodies in
many different ways. Several systems have developed from different
philosophical backgrounds. A common understanding is that wherever
dynamic energies meet together in nature they form spinning circular
patterns, or vortices. The Vedic seers of ancient India also perceived similar
energy vortices within the energy of the human body. Wherever two or
more channels of subtle energy met, there was a vortex, which they named
chakra, meaning wheel.

Where major energy flows coincided on the midline of the body in the front
of the spinal column, there the seers of India saw seven main chakras that
seemed to mirror both health and spiritual well being. These seven chakras
were like multi-dimensional gateways that would allow the individual to
access different experiences and states of consciousness. The use of
visualisation, sound, chant, meditation and exercise to activate, cleanse and
integrate these seven chakras became an important part of spiritual practice
especially in the Himalayan regions of India, Nepal and Tibet.

Many of the original Vedic texts discuss the development of psychic skills
and supernatural powers as a natural result of the spiritual exercises.
Modern translations tended to emphasise the development of the higher
chakras, echoing the desire to go beyond or escape from the bonds of the
physical world. This false division into lower, mundane and higher, spiritual
chakras misses the continually reiterated point in the original texts that all
chakras are of equal practical value both in everyday life and in spiritual
development.

Because they cannot be seen by normal means, the chakras and their related
system of subtle channels, are represented by diagrams and other

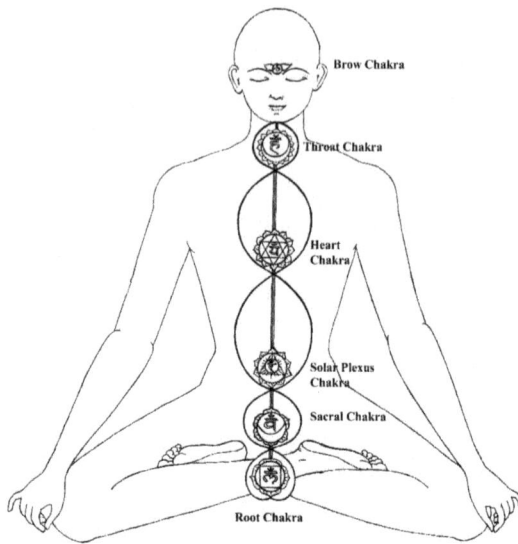

symbolic maps of the body. This is necessary to clarify the relationship of the subtle centres to physical organs and structures with which we are familiar. However, it can also lead to a very static, inflexible and two-dimensional view of what is an elegant, dynamic, ever-changing interaction of energies. Being non-physical, influencing matter but not consisting of matter, chakras are not bound by the laws of matter.

Physical Correspondences

Near each chakra, echoing its function, is one of the main endocrine glands in the body, as well as a concentration of nerves known as a plexus, and concentrations of blood vessels and lymph nodes. As the correspondences are not always linear, some discrepancy sometimes creeps into different systems of comparison, though there is general agreement of the relationships.

The Root Chakra

The first, or root, chakra is located at the base of the spine. In some systems the base is related to the testicles, in others, to the adrenal glands. Although physically a long way from the base, the adrenal glands reflect the survival instinct of this chakra. The coccygeal plexus is the name given to the concentration of nerves in this area. This chakra is linked to the colour red in the comtemporary rainbow system and yellow in the Vedic system.

The Sacral Chakra

The second or sacral chakra, sometimes called the sex chakra, is located in the lower abdomen, between the navel and the pubic bone. It is related to the sacral vertebrae in the spine, the sacral plexus of nerves and the sex glands - the ovaries and testicles. The chakra is associated with emotions and sensuality. This chakra is linked to the colour orange in the rainbow system and white in the Vedic system.

The Solar Plexus Chakra

The third chakra is known as the solar plexus located on the front of the body between the bottom of the ribcage (diaphragm) and the navel. It is concerned with personal energy and power. The glands associated with this centre are the adrenals and the pancreas. The solar plexus chakra is named after the complex of nerves located here and is connected to the lumbar vertebrae of the spine. This chakra is linked to the colour yellow in the rainbow system and red in the Vedic system.

The Heart Chakra

The fourth chakra is the heart, located in the centre of the chest, associated with the thoracic vertebrae of the spine. The related gland is the thymus, a small gland above the heart, vital for growth and maintenance of the immune system. Two nerve centres are located here - the pulmonary plexus and the cardiac plexus. This chakra deals with love and relationship. This chakra is linked to the colour green in both the rainbow and Vedic systems

The Throat Chakra

The fifth chakra is the throat, located near the cervical vertebrae and the base of the throat. It manifests communications and creativity. The thyroid and parathyroid glands (controlling metabolic rate and minerals levels) and the pharyngeal plexus can be found here. This chakra is linked to the colour blue in both the rainbow and Vedic systems

The Brow Chakra

The sixth chakra is the brow, in the centre of the forehead. This is linked to the pineal gland that maintains cycles of activity and rest, and the carotid plexus of nerves. The brow directs intuition, insight and imagination. This chakra is linked to the colour indigo in the rainbow system.

The Crown Chakra

The seventh chakra, the crown, is located just above the top of the head, though it influences all the higher brain functions. It is connected to the pituitary, the master controlling gland for the whole endocrine system. The entire cerebral cortex is influenced by this centre. The crown is associated with knowledge and understanding. This chakra is linked to the colour violet in the rainbow system.

The Subtle Bodies

The chakra system clearly defines different functions and uses of energy in the body. Because of its simplicity and flexibility working with the chakras has become one of the main techniques in healing. What is generally known as the human aura has been identified as a series of interrelated but discrete zones called the subtle bodies. There is less consensus on the exact structure and number of these energy bodies than with the chakra system.

Most cultures define the non-physical bodies in one way or another. Some have two or three, others have five or seven. It can be confusing to try to make sense of different systems, especially as the same names are sometimes used to refer to different things. All subtle systems, be they the chakra, subtle body, meridian or physical are to some extent models and interpretations of how things really are. Each system acts as a guide or map to help us but each is on a different scale. So long as we don't try to use more than one map at any one time we shall find our way perfectly well. Mixing scales, using different systems simultaneously, will tend to confuse the outcome.

The subtle body system can be thought of as different aspects of the individual as seen from particular perspectives and different vibrational rates. Each layer or level is as much "Us" as our physical self but is not made up of solid matter. In much the same way as a normal photograph shows the external features of a person, an ultra-sound scan shows the internal organs and an x-ray photograph shows only the solid and bony tissues of the body, the subtle bodies represent finer, deeper and more subtle qualities of the self.

Described here is a model of seven subtle bodies, each level extending further from the physical body and constituted of finer energy material. It is important to remember that each succeeding level interpenetrates all the previous levels, including the physical, so that there is a continuous, dynamic and complex interaction between them.

The Etheric Body

The etheric body is the closest to the physical, and indeed it is considered to be the energetic blueprint upon which the cells and organs are built. It contains an exact energetic replica of the body with organs and structures the same. When imbalance and weakness occur in the etheric they will eventually manifest on the physical level, so in this respect the etheric body is the last line of defence against disease. Clairvoyant sight describes a blue or blue-grey web of ever-moving energy that extends a little way from the body. The meridian system is believed to be integrated with the etheric body or to act as the interface between etheric and physical.

Giving healing energy to the etheric body will greatly accelerate the repair of physical tissues and may prevent other imbalances from gravitating onto the physical body. The etheric levels are those that often tend to become misaligned from the physical body after shock and trauma. If this mismatch can't correct itself the physical body loses some of its organisational flexibility and this can allow disease states to take hold. Such etheric body dislocation may be the reason why in so many cases a serious period of illness follows a few months after significant shock. Any period of illness or recuperation would benefit from work in this area.

The Emotional Body

The emotional body is the container of feelings. It roughly follows the body's outline but extends further than the etheric. It has no fixed structure and is composed of coloured clouds of energy in continual flux, altering with mood and emotional state. This field is often the aura of colours that sensitives can perceive around a person. The emotional body holds our emotional and psychological stability and our sensitivity to those around us. This body is sometimes called the lower astral, or astral body, which can lead to a confusion with the fourth level, here called the astral. The emotional body is the closest vibratory level to the etheric and contains the volatile and ever-changing energy of our moods. We might think that the environment influences our emotions. Emotion is the weather within us.

For such ephemeral feelings, emotions can play an enormous part in our health and well-being. Each nuance of mood affects the physical body chemistry and even the quality of life-energy that we are able to use. Emotional balance is not an unfeeling, neutral state but a centre point to which the system can return between the extremes of happiness and sorrow. Without this fulcrum/balance/axis as a natural resting place, the emotions can get stuck in a mode of functioning that is inappropriate and deleterious to the body as a whole. Holding on to any particular sort of emotional energy disrupts the whole body weather system.

The Mental Body

The mental body is associated with thoughts and mental processes. It has greater structure than the emotional body and is usually perceived as bright yellow, expanding around the head during mental concentration. Thought patterns exist here as bright shapes coloured with emotion. It is in the mental body that we interpret information according to the belief structures that we have developed since birth.

It has quite distinct and discreet properties. The emotional body reacts, the mental body records, categorises and files these reactions. From birth it constructs how we understand the world and the way it seems to work. It uses all forms of information available to allow the individual to figure out what is going on. The mental body creates our core beliefs and then attaches all other experiences around these central "truths". Unfortunately, the core structures are created very early in life when the tendency is to believe everything we hear and often drastically misinterpret events and the actions of others. Because these structures are so fundamental to our self-image they can be difficult for us to see. Core beliefs can exist in complete contradiction to each other so that when a certain issue arises in life, the opposite pictures of reality can create enormous stress in the body. This stress very often translates into muscular tension and physical rigidity. Easing mental body issues can allow relaxation at many different levels from posture to tolerance of others' beliefs, to flexibility in problem-solving and finding positive options.

The Astral Body

The astral body is the fourth layer. Resembling the emotional body but with clouds of finer and more subtle colouring, this energy layer contains the essence of our personality. It is the boundary layer between the current individual personality and a more collective spiritual awareness, and is concerned with relationship, particularly the sense of encompassing humanity. It is the container that allows us to recognise ourselves as unique beings located in time and space. The astral body filters and tones down all other sources of energy and information so as not to swamp individual consciousness. It can act as a gateway both into physical manifestation and outward towards expanded and collective levels of awareness. Weakness at this level can create great confusion in the perception of reality as the normal constraints of physical reality break down. Too closed an astral body, on the other hand, prevents useful information on other dimensions of energy from integrating into everyday consciousness, which can lead to feelings of unaccountable isolation and loss of direction.

The three remaining subtle bodies are less often described and their functions are not so clearly defined. They certainly are composed of very fine energy.

The fifth layer is sometimes called the **Causal Body**, which links the personality to the collective unconscious and is the doorway to higher levels of consciousness. It patterns the experiences and lessons we have chosen to learn in life. The Causal Body can be seen, by analogy, as the projector that puts our own image onto the screen of physical existence.

The **Soul or Celestial Body** is the sixth subtle level. It seems to focus fine levels of universal energy and is related to the idea of the "Higher Self".

The **Spiritual Body** is the seventh subtle body. It is the container and integrator of all other subtle energies. It has access to all universal energies but maintains the individuality of each being. As the finest level that we know of it is all-embracing, encompassing our whole existence in and outside of time and space.

The Meridians and their Emotional connotations

One simple way of understanding some of the main functions of the meridians is to associate them with emotional states. Thus a positive emotion will energise or strengthen a meridian, whilst its corresponding negative emotional expression will tend to reduce the energy in the meridian. In this way it is possible to identify some of the underlying emotional energy causing disruption to the system. John Diamond, a pioneering kinesiologist, has discovered the attributions of the meridians and emotional states.

Central Meridian (Conception Vessel) [CV1-CV24]
Begins at the perineum and ends just below the lower lip.
Positive emotions are: love, faith, gratitude, trust, courage.
Negative states are: hate, envy, fear.

Governing Vessel[GV1-GV28]
Begins at the tail bone, rises up the spine over the head to the centre of the upper lip. There are no specific emotional states listed except as for the central meridian.

Gallbladder Meridian [GB1-GB44]
Begins at the outer edge of the eye and finishes at the outer end of the fourth toe.
Positive emotions are: reaching out with love and forgiveness, and adoration.
Negative emotions are: rage, fury and wrath.

Liver Meridian [Liv1-Liv14]
Starts at the outside of the big toe and ends at the bottom of the ribcage below the sternum.
Positive emotions are: happiness and cheerfulness,
Negative emotion is: unhappiness.

Bladder Meridian.[B1-B67]

Begins at the inner canthus of the eye (against the bridge of the nose), and ends on the outer edge of the little toe.

Positive emotions are: peace and harmony.

Negative emotions are: restlessness, impatience and frustration.

Kidney Meridian.[K1-K27]

Begins at the ball of the foot and ends where the collar and breast-bones meet.

Positive states relate to: sexual assuredness,

Negative states to: sexual indecision.

Large Intestine (Colon) Meridian [LI1-LI20]

Begins on the inner end of the index fingers and ends on the face by the outer edge of the nostrils.

Positive emotions are: self-worth, acceptance.

The negative state is: guilt.

Lung Meridian [Lu1- Lu11]

Begins just below the corocoid process on the shoulder and ends on the inner end of the thumb.

Positive emotions are: humility, tolerance and modesty.

Negative states are: disdain, contempt and prejudice.

Stomach Meridian [St1- St45]

Begins below the eye at the inner edge of the orbit, and finishes at the outer end of the second toe.

Positive emotions are: contentment and tranquillity.

Negative states are: disappointment, disgust, bitterness, greed, nausea, hunger, emptiness.

Spleen Meridian [Sp1- Sp21]

Begins at the inner edge of the big toe and ends at the side of the chest just below nipple level.

Positive emotions are: faith and confidence about the future and security.

Negative emotions are: realistic anxieties about the future.

Circulation-Sex Meridian.(Pericardium, Heart Protector) [Cx1- Cx9]

Begins at the outer edge of the nipple and finishes at the inside end of the middle finger.

Positive states are: relaxation, generosity, renouncing the past, letting go.

Negative states are: regret, remorse, jealousy, sexual tension, stubbornness.

Triple Warmer Meridian (Triple Heater) [Tw1- Tw23]

Begins at the outside end of the ring finger (third) and ends at the outer edge of the eyebrow.

Positive emotions are: elation, hope, lightness, buoyancy.

Negative states are: loneliness, despondency, grief, hopelessness, despair and depression.

Heart Meridian[H1- H9]

Begins at the forward edge of the armpit and ends on the inner edge of the little finger.

Positive emotions are: love and forgiveness.

Negative emotion is: anger.

Small Intestine Meridian [SI1- SI19]

Begins at the outer end of the little fingertip and ends at the upper edge of the ear in a small hollow of the cheek.

The positive state is: joy,

The negative states are: sadness and sorrow.

Brief Colour Correspondences

RED   keyword: *energy*
Physical - activating, energising, heating, circulation, prana, blood, practicality
Emotional - assertiveness, passion, anger
Mental - initiative, daring, penetrating
Spiritual - grounding, protecting, manifestation of spiritual energies in the world
Chakra: Root ('Base')
Meridians: Triple Warmer (Triple Heater); Circulation/Sex,
                Pericardium (Heart Protector); Heart,

ORANGE   keyword: *recovery*
Physical - for shock or trauma at any level , stagnant energies, detoxification, creativity
Emotional - fun, sense of play, pleasure, sensuality
Mental - artistry, creativity
Spiritual - repairs the etheric template, centres energy, brings energy into the present
Chakra: Sacral or Second
Meridians: Large Intestine; Gall Bladder

YELLOW   keyword : *discrimination*
Physical - ability to recognise and identify what is of use to the body and what is not.
Emotional - joy, contentment, happiness
Mental - clarity, memory, study, intellect
Spiritual - wisdom, Self-knowledge
Chakra: Solar plexus
Meridians: Stomach, Spleen; Kidney, Bladder; Small Intestine.

GREEN   keyword: *calm*
Physical - attunement to Nature, growth, expansion and contraction
Emotional - love, balance, caring, sharing
Mental - independence, space, freedom
Spiritual - personal direction or Path
Chakra: Heart
Meridians: Lung, Large Intestine, Liver

BLUE   keyword: *communication*
Physical - cooling, flow of communication
Emotional - detachment, peace, loyalty
Mental - expression, quiet
Spiritual - subtle communication
Chakra: Throat
Meridians: Stomach, Spleen

INDIGO   keyword: *perception*
Physical - very cooling
Emotional - very detached, almost cold
Mental - perceptions, intuition, very quietening, ability to discern patterns in life
Spiritual - far memory, controls psychic current in the body
Chakra: Ajna or Brow
Meridians: All

VIOLET   keywords: *release of full potential*
Physical - balance of energies in the head, overall healer
Emotional - empathy, sensitivity
Mental - imagination, inspiration, balances logic and emotion
Spiritual - integrates to help link to full potential, co-creation
Chakra: Crown
Meridians: all, but especially, Bladder, Gall Bladder

PINK   keyword: *love*
Physical - calms aggressive situations
Emotional - self-acceptance, self-tolerance, self-love etc.
Mental - trust, compassion
Spiritual - understanding the underlying unity within the diversity of creation
Chakras: Heart, Sacral
Meridians: Large Intestine, Kidney, Heart

WHITE   keyword: *transformation*
All levels: Cleanses on every level and cuts away unwanted debris creating clarity and transformation. Creates space to develop and change. New beginnings, rebirth, purification.

MAGENTA   keyword : *compassion*
Physical - ability to release and change
Emotional - stabilises emotions, giving and receiving
Mental - adaptability, flexibility
Spiritual - heals and stabilises all subtle bodies
Chakras: Sacral; Above the Crown
Meridians: Triple Warmer, Heart Protector

Guidelines for Using Essences

Our own tree essences, *Green Man Essences* are handmade using traditional methods. The energy signatures are held in water and preserved in 23% ABV.

All our essences are provided at ***stock*** level which allows you to dilute 3-7 drops in a dosage bottle containing a water or a 60/40 mix of alcohol (about 22.5% ABV).

Flower and vibrational essences have traditionally been taken by mouth, that is, a few drops placed in a small glass of water or in a small dropper bottle full of water. A few drops can be placed under the tongue.

Some people find the following methods useful:

· Putting a drop on the pulse points (wrists, throat, neck, forehead, soles of the feet)
· Putting a few drops on your hands, rub them together and then sweep around the body, a few centimetres above the skin or clothes
· Rub a drop of essence between your palms and then cup your hands near your nose and breathe in the essence as it evaporates
· Put a few drops into an atomiser or sprayer containing water. Spray around the body or room
· Add a few drops to some massage oil
· Add drops to your bathwater
· An essence can be very effective when placed upon a specific chakra or meridian point.

A good guideline for using essences is 3 or 4 times a day, or you can determine the frequency or method by dowsing or muscle-testing.

Lightning Source UK Ltd.
Milton Keynes UK
UKHW020626290520
364047UK00009B/718